Keto Slow Cooker Cookbook

50 Healthy and Delicious Ketogenic Recipes for your Slow Cooker

By Susan Campbell

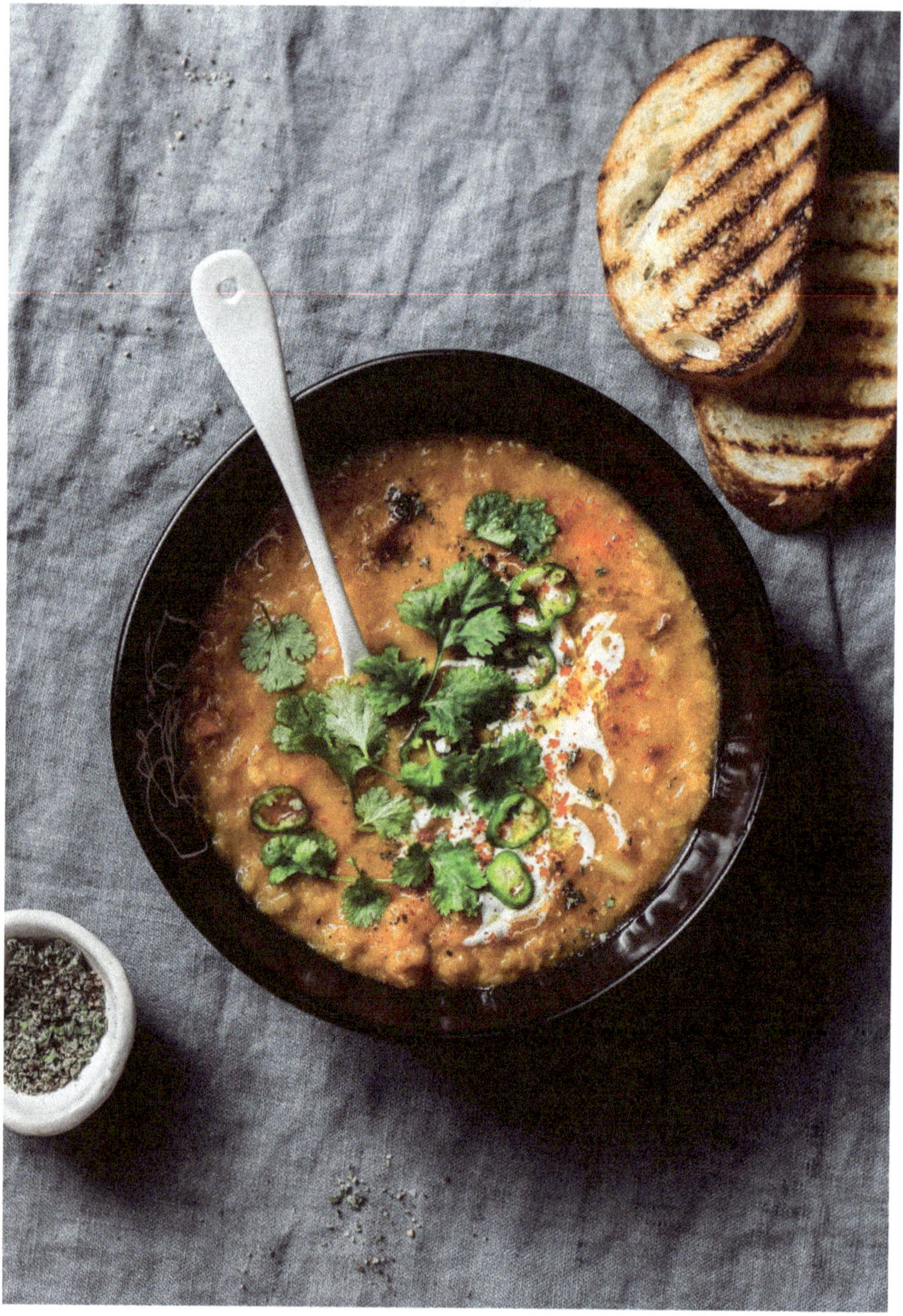

Table of Contents

Chapter 1: Breakfast

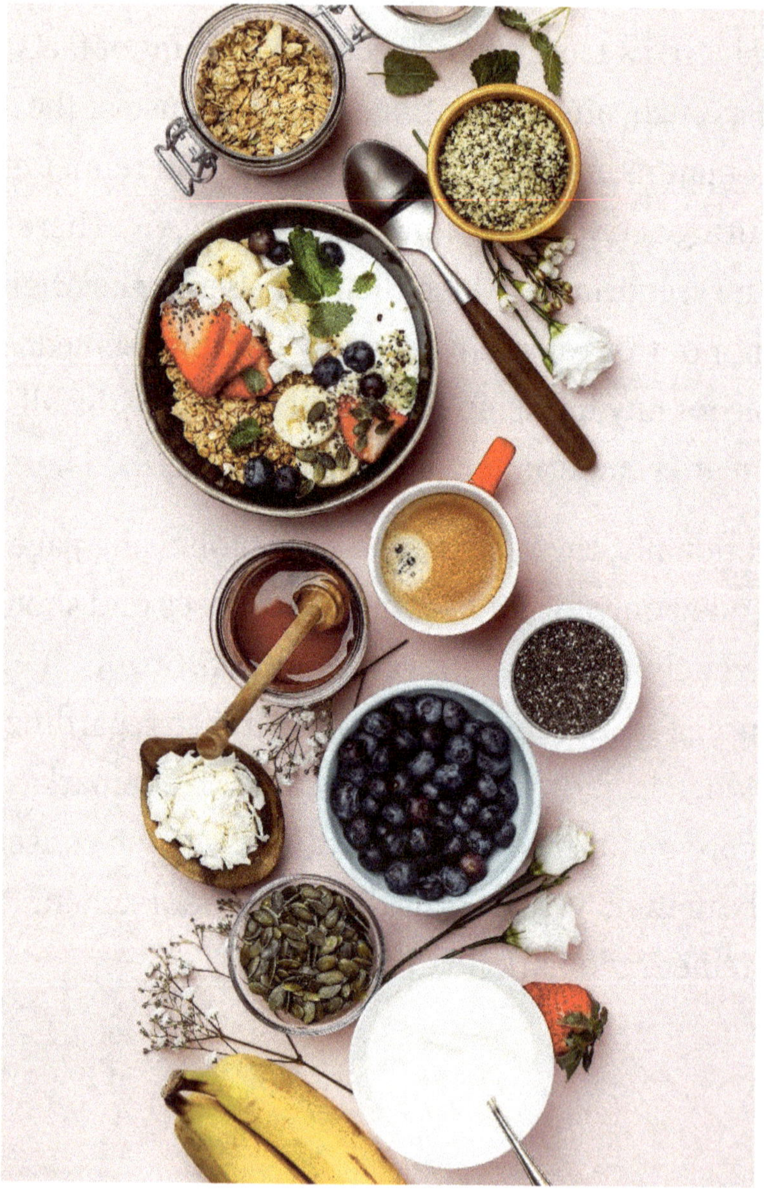

Vanilla Pumpkin Bread

Preparation: 10 min | Cooking: 2 h | Servings: 2

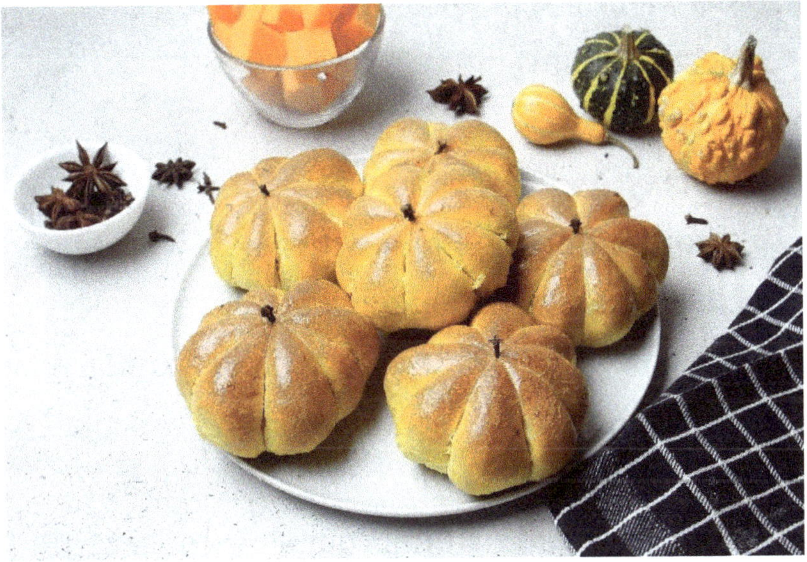

Ingredients

- Cooking spray
- ½ cup white flour
- ½ cup whole wheat flour
- ½ teaspn baking soda
- A pinch of cinnamon powder
- 2 tsps olive oil
- 2 tsps maple syrup
- 1 egg

- ½ tbsp milk
- ½ teaspn vanilla extract
- ½ cup pumpkin puree
- 2 tsps walnuts, chopped
- 2 tsps chocolate chips

Directions

1. In a bowl, mix white flour with whole wheat flour, baking soda, and cinnamon and stir.
2. Add maple syrup, olive oil, egg, milk, vanilla extract, pumpkin puree, walnuts, and chocolate chips and stir well.
3. Grease a loaf pan that fits your slow cooker with cooking spray, pour pumpkin bread, transfer to your cooker and cook on High for 2 h.
4. Slice bread, divide between plates, and serve.
5. Enjoy!

Nutrition: calories 200, Fat: 3, Fiber: 5, Carbs: 8, Protein: 4

Apple, Avocado, and Mango Bowls

Preparation: 10 min | Cooking: 2 h | Servings: 2

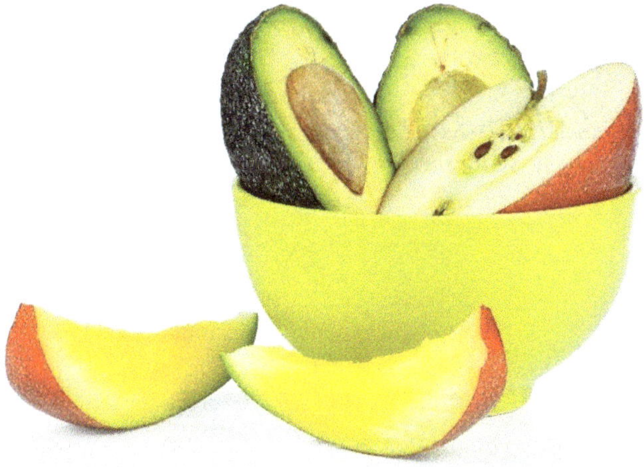

Ingredients:

- 1 cup avocado, peeled, pitted, and cubed
- 1 cup mango, peeled and cubed
- 1 apple, cored and cubed
- 2 tsps brown sugar
- 1 cup heavy cream
- 1 tbsp lemon juice

Directions:

1. In your slow cooker, combine the avocado with the mango and the other ingredients, toss gently, put the lid on and cook on Low for 2 h.
2. Divide the mix into bowls and serve.

Nutrition: Calories: 60, Fat: 1, Fiber: 2, Carbs: 20, Protein: 1

Vanilla Pancakes

Preparation: 15 min | Cooking: 2 h | Servings: 6

Ingredients:

- 1 cup coconut flour
- 2 eggs, beaten
- 1 teaspn baking powder
- 1 tbsp vanilla extract
- 1 tbsp ghee
- ½ cup almond milk
- ¾ teaspn salt
- ¼ teaspn nutmeg

Directions:

1. Whisk the eggs with the coconut flour and baking powder in the mixing bowl.
2. Add vanilla extract and ghee.
3. Then add milk, salt, and nutmeg.
4. Stir the pancake mixture carefully until smooth.
5. Pour the pancake batter into the slow cooker and close the lid.
6. Cook the pancake for 2 h on High.

7. When the pancake is cooked, cut it into servings and serve.
8. Enjoy!

Nutrition: calories: 173, fat: 10.4, fiber: 8.5, carbs: 15.3, protein: 5

Cheesy Turmeric Eggs

Preparation: 10 min | Cooking: 1 h 30 min | Servings: 4

Ingredients:

- 4 eggs, beaten
- ¾ teaspn turmeric
- 1 tbsp butter, melted
- 3 tsps almond milk, unsweetened
- 2 oz of Parmesan, grated

Directions:

1. Whisk the eggs and with the turmeric, butter, and almond milk.
2. Pour the mix into the slow cooker.
3. Cook the eggs for 1 h on High.
4. Scramble the eggs with a spatula and sprinkle with the grated cheese.
5. Cook the omelet for 30 min more on Low.
6. Enjoy!

Nutrition: calories: 161, fat: 13, fiber: 0.3, carbs: 5, protein: 10.4

Egg, Spinach, and Ham Breakfast Casserole

Preparation: 10 min | Cooking: 1 hour and 30 min | Servings: 6

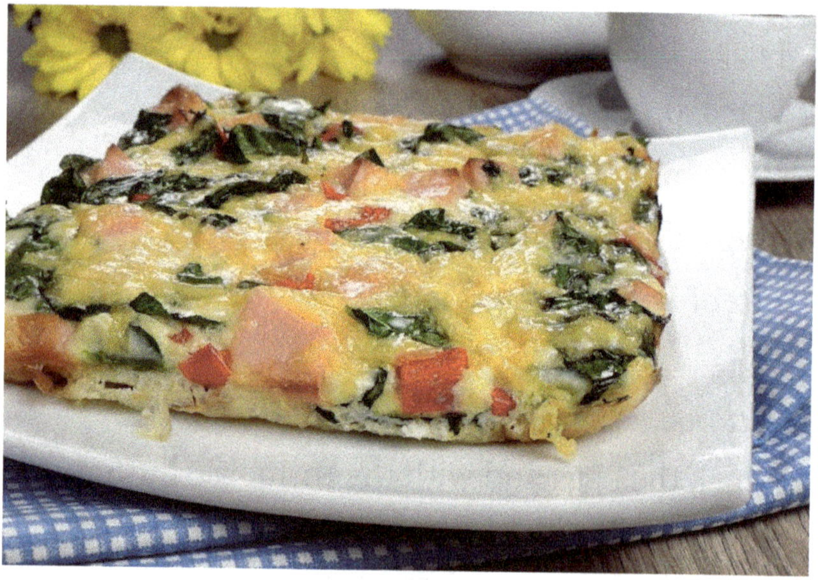

Ingredients:

- Large eggs - 6
- Salt - ½ teaspn
- Black pepper - ¼ teaspn
- Milk - ¼ cup
- Greek yogurt - ½ cup
- Thyme - ½ teaspn

- Onion powder - ½ teaspn
- Garlic powder - ½ teaspn
- Diced mushrooms - ⅓ cup
- Baby spinach (packed) – 1 cup
- Shredded pepper jack cheese – 1 cup
- Ham, diced – 1 cup

Directions:

1. Mix eggs, salt, pepper, milk, yogurt, thyme, onion powder, garlic powder properly in a bowl.
2. Add mushrooms, spinach, cheese, ham, and stir.
3. Now take a 6-quart slow cooker and spray with non-stick cooking spray.
4. Pour egg mixture into the cooker and put on slow.
5. Cover and cook on high for 90-120 min until eggs arc appropriately set.
6. Slice and serve for breakfast or dinner.

Nutrition: Calories: 155.6 Total Fat: 8.7 g Cholesterol 86.1 mg Sodium 758.8 mg Total Carbs: 2.5 g Dietary fiber 0.3 g Protein:15.6 g

Chapter 2: Lunch

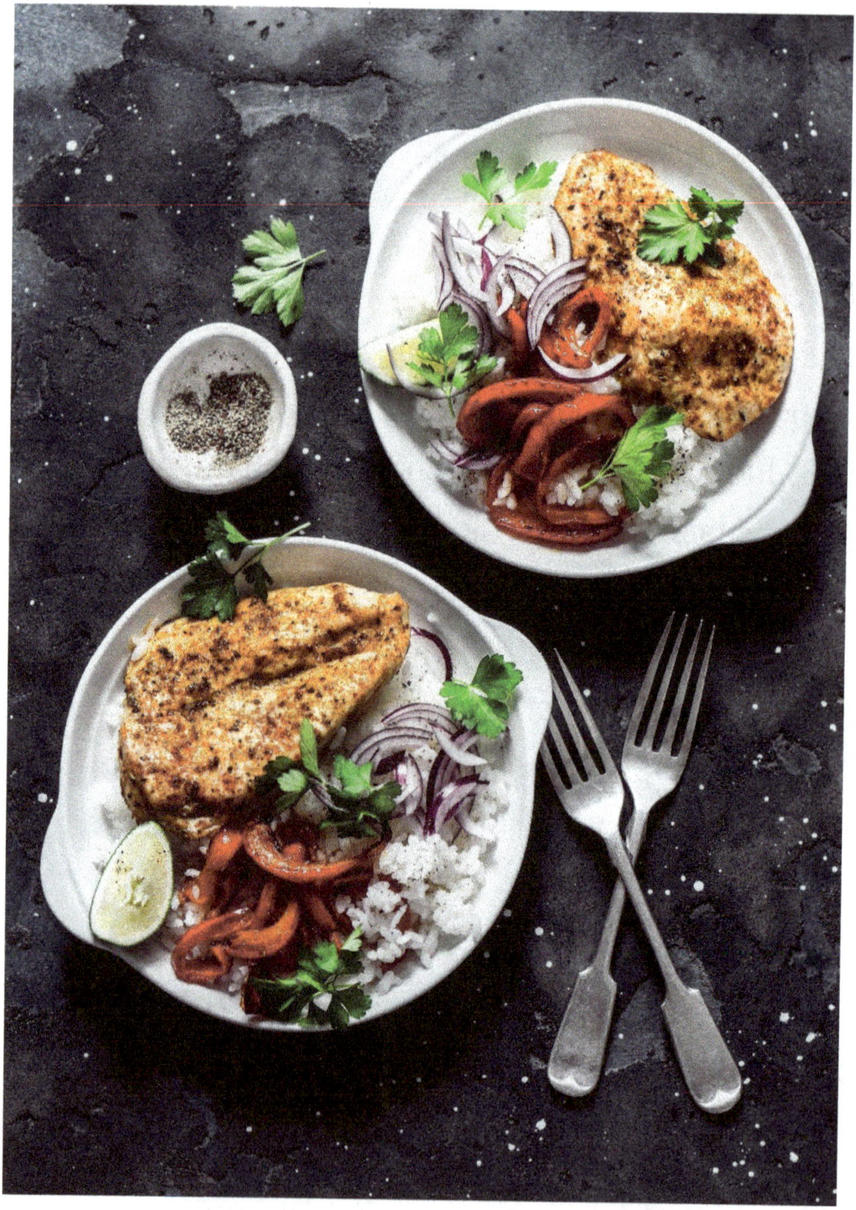

Sloppy Joes

Servings: 4 | Preparation: 5 min | Cooking: 6 hours

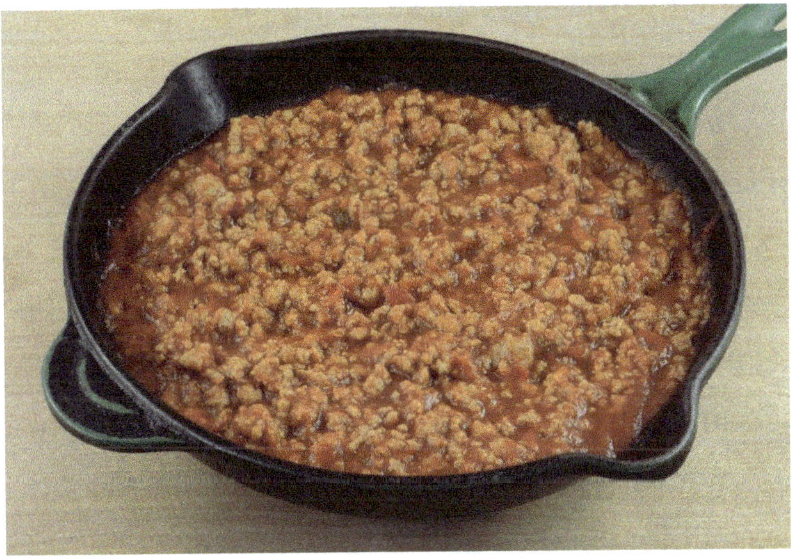

Ingredients:

- 1 pound ground beef, grass-fed
- 1|4 cup chopped green bell pepper
- 1|4 cup chopped white onion
- 1|2 teaspn garlic powder
- 1 teaspn salt
- ½ teaspn ground black pepper
- 1 teaspn yellow mustard paste
- 1 tbsp avocado oil

- 1|2 cup tomato ketchup, sugar-free
- 3 teaspns swerve sweetener
- ½ cup beef broth
- Grated parmesan cheese for topping

Directions:

1. Place a large skillet pan over medium-high heat, add oil and when hot, add ground beef, onion, and garlic powder and cook for 5 to 7 min or until beef is nicely browned.
2. Drain fat from the pan, spoon beef mixture into a 6-quars slow cooker, add remaining ingredients except for cheese and stir until mixed.
3. Plug in the slow cooker, shut with lid and cook for 4 to 6 hours at low heat setting or until cooked through.
4. Spoon beef in a lettuce cup or roasted mushroom cap, top with parmesan cheese and serve.

Nutrition: Net Carbs: 2.5g; Calories: 451; Total Fat: 29g; Saturated Fat: 13.5g; Protein: 38.3g; Carbs: 9g; Fiber: 6.5g; Sugar: 2.6g Total Fat: 58%; Protein: 34%; Carbs: 8%;

Bologneseervings: 4 | Preparation: 5 min | Cooking: 4 hours

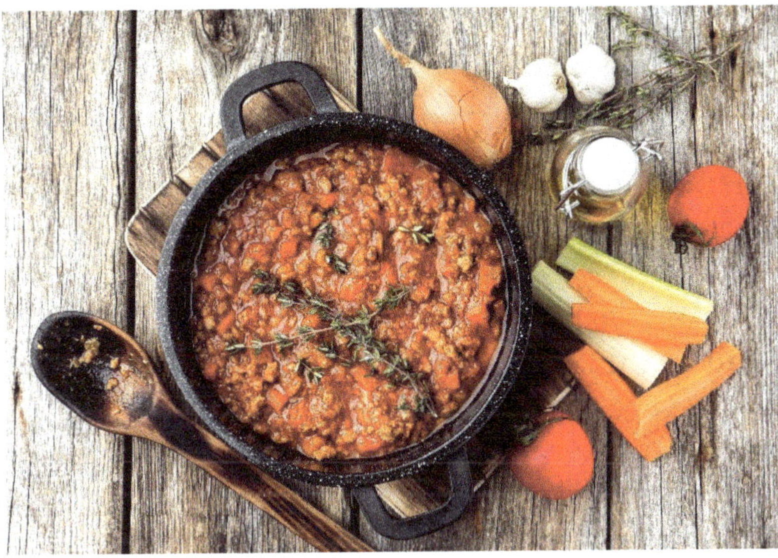

Ingredients:

- 1 pound ground beef, grass-fed
- 14.5 ounce diced tomatoes
- 1 teaspn onion powder
- 1 teaspn salt
- ½ teaspn ground black pepper
- 1 teaspn Italian seasoning
- 3 tsps avocado oil
- 8-ounce tomato sauce
- 3 bay leaves

Directions:

1. Place a large skillet pan over medium heat, add beef, season with onion powder and Italian seasoning and cook for 7 to 10 min or until nicely browned.
2. Then drain fat from the pan, transfer beef to a 6-quart slow cooker and add remaining ingredients.
3. Plug in the slow cooker, stir all the ingredients until just mix, then shut with lid and cook for 4 hours at low heat setting or 8 hours at high heat setting until cooked.
4. Serve straightaway.

Nutrition: Net Carbs: 4g; Calories: 411.5; Total Fat: 28.8g; Saturated Fat: 17g; Protein: 31.9g; Carbs: 6g; Fiber: 2g; Sugar: 5g Total Fat: 63%; Protein: 31%; Carbs: 6%;

Zuppa Toscana Soup

Servings: 10 | Preparation: 5 min | Cooking: 8 hours and 10 min

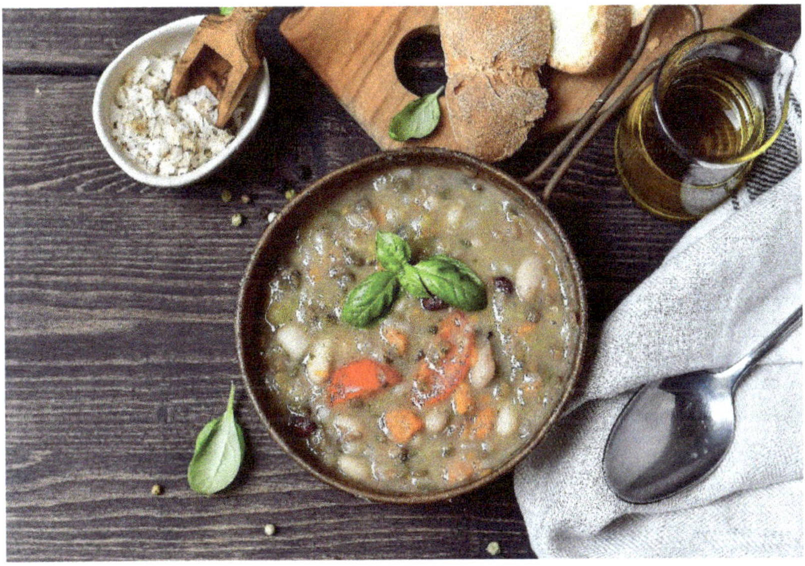

Ingredients:

- 1 pound ground Italian sausage, grass-fed
- 1 large cauliflower head, cut into small florets
- 3 cups chopped kale
- ½ cup diced white onion
- 1 ½ teaspn minced garlic
- 1 teaspn salt
- ½ teaspn ground black pepper

- ¼ teaspn crushed red pepper flakes
- 1 tbsp avocado oil
- 36 ounces chicken stock
- ½ cup heavy cream

Directions:

1. Place a large skillet pan over medium heat, add sausage and cook for 7 to 10 min or until nicely brown.
2. Drain fat from pan and transfer sausage to a 6-quart slow cooker.
3. Add oil into the skillet and when hot, add onion and cook for 3 to 4 min or until beginning to soften.
4. Transfer onions to the slow cooker cooked and remaining ingredients except for heavy cream and stir until mixed.
5. Plug in the slow cooker, then shut with lid and cook for 8 hours at low heat setting or 4 hours at high heat setting until cooked through.
6. When done, stir in heavy cream and serve immediately.

Nutrition: Net Carbs: 3g; Calories: 255; Total Fat: 19g; Saturated Fat: 7g; Protein: 14g; Carbs: 7g; Fiber: 4g; Sugar: 3g Total Fat: 68%; Protein: 22%; Carbs: 10%;

Cheeseburger Meatloaf

Servings: 8 | Preparation: 5 min | Cooking: 8 hours

Ingredients:

- 2 pounds ground beef, grass-fed
- 1 teaspn garlic powder
- 2 teaspns salt
- 1 small white onion, peeled and diced
- 2 eggs
- 1/2 cup grated Parmesan cheese
- 1/2 cup cheddar cheese, cut into cubes

Directions:

1. Place all the ingredients in a large bowl, except for cheddar cheese and stir until just mixed, don't over mix.
2. Then fold in cheese cubes and shape mixture into meatloaf.
3. Plug in 6-quarts slow cooker, then line with aluminum foil, add meatloaf and shut with lid.
4. Cook meatloaf for 7 to 8 hours at low heat setting or 4 to 5 hours at high heat setting or until cooked.

5. When done, take out meatloaf using aluminum foil, rest for 5 min, then slice evenly and serve.

Nutrition: Net Carbs: 2g; Calories: 279; Total Fat: 19g; Saturated Fat: 7g; Protein: 25g; Carbs: 2g; Fiber: 0g; Sugar: 1g Total Fat: 61%; Protein: 36%; Carbs: 3%;

Chorizo and Peppers

Servings: 8 | Preparation: 5 min | Cooking: 10 hours

Ingredients:

- 2 pounds pasture-raised chorizo sausage, casings removed and crumbled
- 2 medium green bell peppers, seeded and chopped
- 2 medium white onion, peeled and chopped
- 2 tsps minced garlic
- 1 ½ tbsp avocado oil
- 6-ounce tomato paste, unsweetened
- 1 cup water
- 1 cup red wine

Directions:

1. Place sausage in a 6-quart slow cooker, crumble it, then add remaining ingredients and stir until combined.
2. Plug in the slow cooker, shut with lid and cook for 8 hours at low heat or until cooked through.
3. Then uncover slow cooker and cook more for 2 hours or until some of the cooking liquid evaporates.

4. Serve straightaway.

Nutrition: Net Carbs: 6g; Calories: 370; Total Fat: 25g; Saturated Fat: 2.4g; Protein: 29g; Carbs: 8g; Fiber: 2g; Sugar: 2.4g Total Fat: 60%; Protein: 31%; Carbs: 9%;

Chapter 3: Red Meat

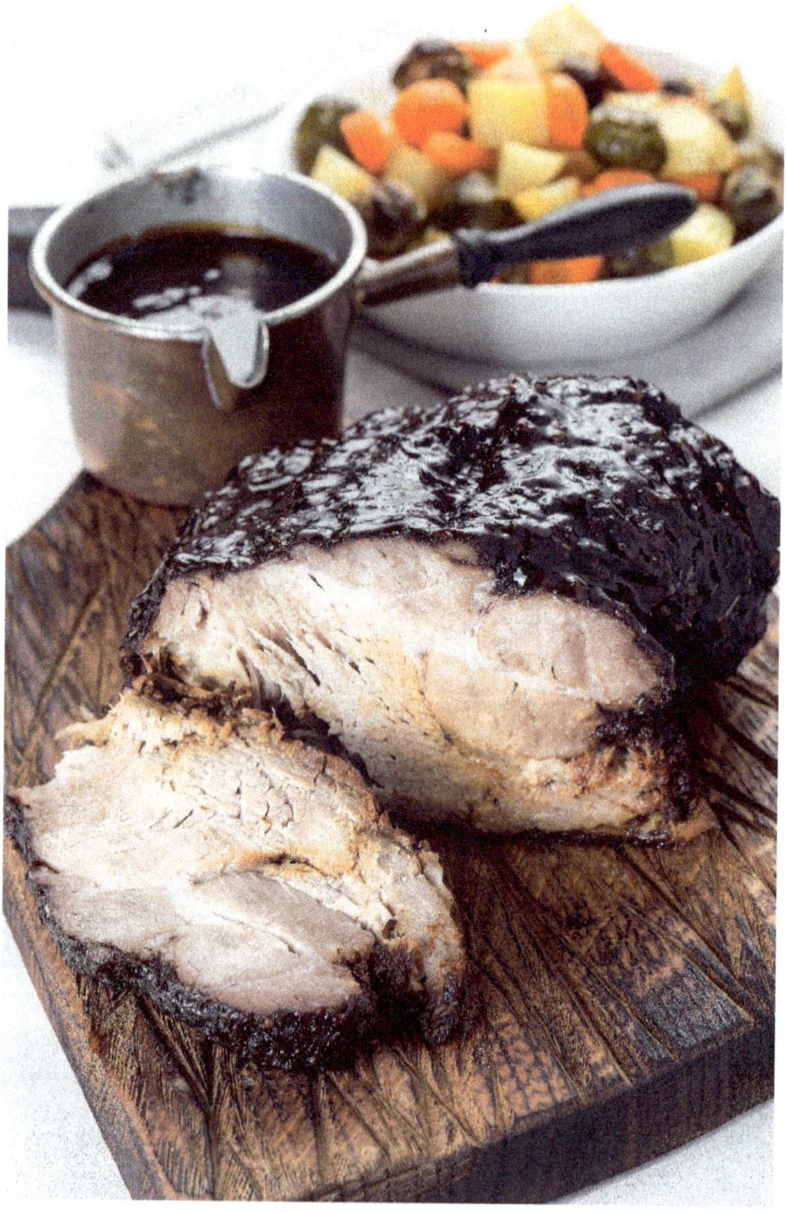

Beef Chuck Roast with Mustard Sauce

Servings: 8 | Preparation: 5 min | Cooking: 8 hours

Ingredients:

- 3 pounds grass-fed beef chuck roast, cut to 1-inch cubes
- 2 stalks of celery, chopped
- 1/2 of a medium onion, peeled and diced
- 1 teaspn garlic powder
- 1 teaspn salt
- 3 tsps mustard paste
- 4-ounce heavy cream

Dircctions:

1. Whisk together garlic, salt, mustard, and cream and pour this mixture into a 6-quart slow cooker.
2. Plug in the slow cooker, add roast, celery, and onion and then shut with lid.
3. Cook for 8 hours at low heat setting or 4 hours at high heat setting or until cooked through.
4. Serve straightaway.

Nutrition: Net Carbs: 0.4g; Calories: 364; Total Fat: 25g; Saturated Fat: 11g; Protein: 33g; Carbs: 1g; Fiber: 0.6g; Sugar: 9g Total Fat: 63%; Protein: 36%; Carbs: 1%;

Taco Soup with Beef

Servings: 6 | Preparation: 5 min | Cooking: 4 hours and 40 min

Ingredients:

- 2-pound grass-fed ground beef
- 1 medium tomato
- ½ of a small white onion
- ½ teaspn minced garlic
- 1 ½ teaspn salt
- 1 teaspn ground black pepper
- 1 teaspn paprika
- 1 teaspn cumin powder
- 1 tbsp avocado oil
- 1/2 cup tomato puree
- 3 1/2 cup chicken broth
- 1 cup cream cheese
- 1 cup shredded cheddar cheese

Directions:

1. Place a large skillet pan over medium heat, add ground beef and cook for 5 min or until seared.

2. Then add onion, garlic, and oil and cook for 5 to 10 min or until beef is cooked completely.
3. Transfer beef into a 6-quart slow cooker, add remaining ingredients except for cheeses and stir until mixed.
4. Plug in the slow cooker, shut with lid and cook for 4 hours at low heat setting or 2 hours at high heat setting.
5. Then stir in cheeses and continue cooking the soup for 30 min.
6. Serve straightaway.

Nutrition: Net Carbs: 4.8g; Calories: 569; Total Fat: 41.2g; Saturated Fat: 15g; Protein: 43g; Carbs: 5.8g; Fiber: 1g; Sugar: 5g Total Fat: 66%; Protein: 30%; Carbs: 4%;

Mexican Shredded Beef

Servings: 10 | Preparation: 5 min | Cooking: 9 hours

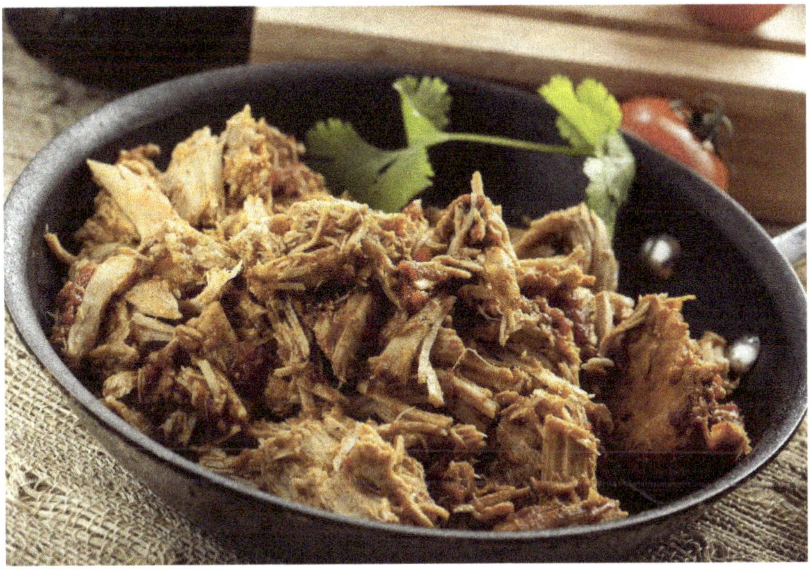

Ingredients:

- 3 pounds grass-fed beef chuck roast
- 1 medium white onion, peeled and diced
- 2 teaspns minced garlic
- 1 teaspn salt
- 1 tbsp red chili powder
- 1/4 teaspn red chili flakes
- 1 teaspn paprika
- 1 teaspn cumin

- 1 teaspn dried oregano
- 2 tsps avocado oil
- 2 tsps tomato paste
- 2 tsps lime juice
- Sour cream for topping

Directions:

1. Prepare spice mix and for this, stir together salt, red chili powder, red chili flakes, paprika, cumin, and oregano.
2. Place onion and garlic in a 6-quart slow cooker, add oil and 2 teaspns of spice mix, along with tomato paste and lime juice and stir until mixed.
3. Season beef roast with remaining spice mix, add to slow cooker on top of onion mixture and shut with lid.
4. Plug in the slow cooker and cook for 7 to 8 hours at a low heat setting or more until cooked through.
5. When done, shred beef with two forks, stir well into the sauce and cook for another 30 to 60 min.
6. Serve straightaway.

Nutrition: Net Carbs: 1g; Calories: 519; Total Fat: 34.6g; Saturated Fat: 14.7g; Protein: 49.3g; Carbs:

2.6g; Fiber: 1.6g; Sugar: 1.6g Total Fat: 60%; Protein: 38%; Carbs: 2%;

Ground Beef Eggplant Casserole

Servings: 12 | Preparation: 5 min | Cooking: 4 hours

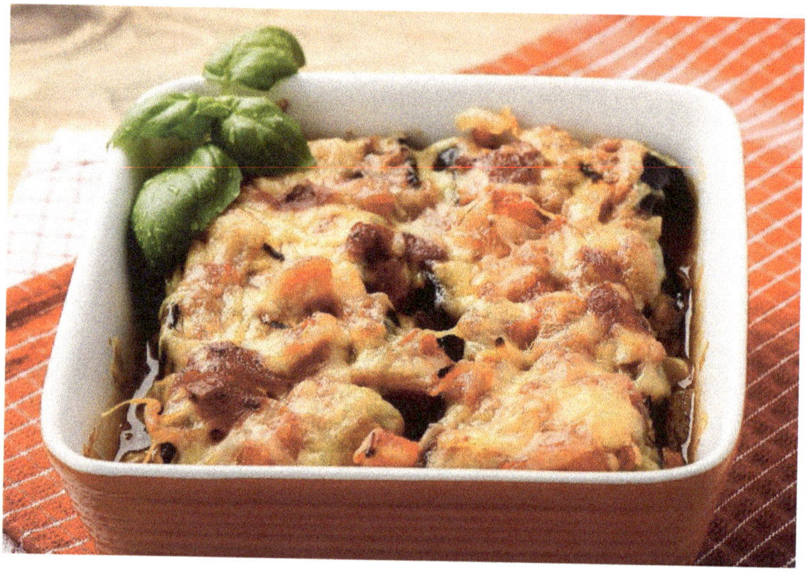

Ingredients:

- 2 pounds ground beef, grass-fed
- 2 cups eggplant cubes
- 28 ounces diced tomatoes
- 2 1/8 teaspn salt
- ½ teaspn ground black pepper
- 2 teaspns mustard
- 2 tsps parsley
- 1 teaspn dried oregano

- 3 tsps avocado oil
- 2 teaspns Worcestershire sauce
- 16 ounces tomato sauce
- 2 cups grated mozzarella cheese

Directions:

1. Place eggplant cubes in a colander, season with 1|8 teaspn salt, toss until mixed and let rest for 30 min.
2. Then transfer eggplants into a large bowl, add oil and toss until well coated.
3. Stir together beef, salt, black pepper, Worcestershire sauce, and mustard, then place in a 6-quarts slow cooker and spread evenly.
4. Top with eggplant pieces, then spread with tomatoes and tomato sauce and sprinkle with parsley and oregano.
5. Plug in the slow cooker, then shut with lid and cook for 3 to 4 hours at low heat setting or 2 to 3 hours at high heat setting.
6. Serve straightaway.

Nutrition: Net Carbs: 3g; Calories: 329; Total Fat: 21.5g; Saturated Fat: 11.2g; Protein: 25.5g; Carbs:

8.2g; Fiber: 5.2g; Sugar: 5.4g Total Fat: 59%; Protein: 31%; Carbs: 10%;

BBQ Beef Brisket

Servings: 6 | Preparation: 5 min | Cooking: 10 hours

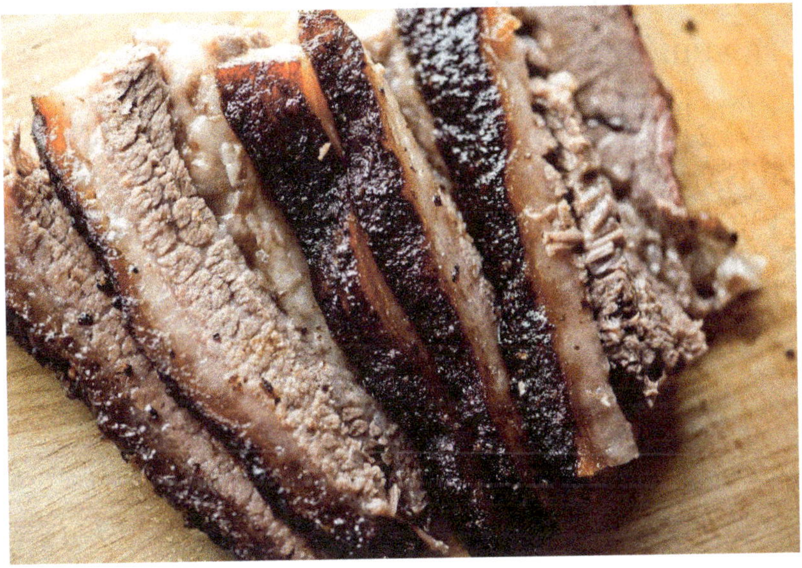

Ingredients:

- 3.5 pounds beef brisket, grass-fed
- 1 teaspn onion powder
- 1 teaspn garlic powder
- 1 teaspn celery salt
- 1 teaspn smoked paprika
- 1/8 teaspn ground black pepper
- 4.5 ounce BBQ sauce, unsweetened
- ¼ cup beef broth

Directions:

1. Place beef in a 6-quart slow cooker, stir together onion powder, garlic powder, salt, and paprika and rub this mixture over beef brisket.
2. Pour in BBQ sauce and beef stock and shut with lid.
3. Plug in the slow cooker and cook beef for 8 to 10 hours at low heat setting or until tender.
4. When done, shred beef with two forks, stir well to coat with sauce and serve.

Nutrition: Net Carbs: 2.2g; Calories: 894.5; Total Fat: 69.5g; Saturated Fat: 29.8g; Protein: 64.8g; Carbs: 2.2g; Fiber: 0g; Sugar: 4g Total Fat: 70%; Protein: 29%; Carbs: 1%;

Autumn Pork Stew

Preparation: 30 min | Cooking: 6 h | Servings: 5

Ingredients:

- 1 eggplant, chopped
- 4 oz of white mushrooms, chopped
- 1 white onion, chopped
- 2 cups water
- ½ teaspn clove
- ½ teaspn salt
- ½ teaspn cayenne pepper
- 8 oz of pork tenderloin

Directions:

1. Place the chopped eggplant, mushrooms, onion, and water in the slow cooker.
2. Chop the pork tenderloin roughly and sprinkle it with the cayenne pepper, salt, and clove.
3. Stir the meat and place it in the slow cooker too.
4. Close the lid and cook the stew for 6 h on Low.
5. When the stew is cooked, let it rest for 20 min.
6. Enjoy!

Nutrition: calories: 232, fat: 5.1, fiber: 4.1, carbs: 8.4, protein: 37.5

Thyme Lamb Chops

Preparation: 20 min | Cooking: 7 h | Servings: 2

Ingredients:

- 8 oz of lamb chops
- 1 teaspn liquid stevia
- 1 teaspn thyme
- 1 tbsp olive oil
- ¼ cup water
- 1 bay leaf
- ¾ teaspn ground cinnamon
- ½ onion, chopped

Directions:

1. Mix the liquid stevia, thyme, olive oil, and ground cinnamon.
2. Rub the lamb chops with the spice mixture.
3. Place the lamb chops in the slow cooker and add chopped onion and water.
4. Add the bay leaf and close the lid.
5. Cook the lamb chops for 7 h on Low.
6. When the meat is cooked, serve it immediately!

Nutrition: calories: 287, fat: 15.4, fiber: 1.4, carbs: 4, protein: 32.3

Garlic Pork Belly

Preparation: 15 min | Cooking: 7 h | Servings: 8

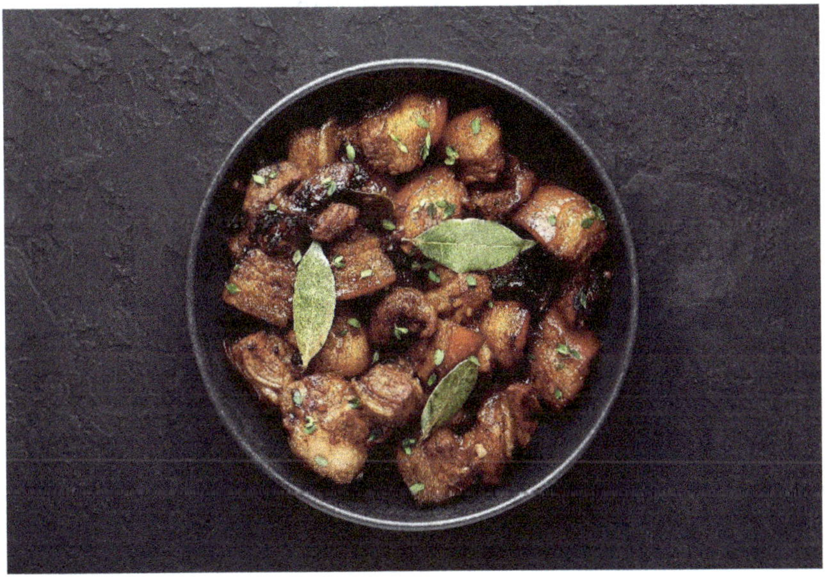

Ingredients:

- 1-pound pork belly
- 4 garlic cloves, peeled
- 1 teaspn peppercorns
- 2 tsps mustard
- ½ teaspn salt
- 1 tbsp butter
- 1 cup water

Directions:

1. Dice the garlic cloves and combine them with the peppercorns and mustard.
2. Add the salt and butter and stir.
3. Rub the pork belly with the prepared mixture well.
4. Place the pork belly in the slow cooker.
5. Add the water and close the lid.
6. Cook the pork belly for 7 h on Low.
7. Slice the cooked pork belly and serve!

Nutrition: calories: 290, fat: 17.5, fiber: 0.5, carbs: 1.7, protein: 27

Paprika Pork Sausages

Preparation: 15 min | Cooking: 2 h | Servings: 4

Ingredients:

- 10 oz of ground pork
- 1 tbsp paprika
- 2 egg yolks
- ½ teaspn salt
- 1 teaspn ground black pepper
- ½ onion, grated
- 1 tbsp almond flour

Directions:

1. Mix the ground pork and egg yolks.
2. Stir the ground pork with a fork until well blended.
3. Add paprika, salt, ground black pepper, and almond flour.
4. Stir the pork mixture and add the grated onion.
5. Stir it well and form medium sausages using your hands.
6. Then place the sausages in the slow cooker.
7. Close the lid and cook for 2 h on High.

8. Then transfer the sausages to the platter and enjoy!

Nutrition: calories: 180, fat: 8.5, fiber: 1.8, carbs: 4.4, protein: 21.9

Asian Chopped Beef

Preparation: 20 min | Cooking: 3 h | Servings: 4

Ingredients:

- 1-pound beef chops
- 2 tsps apple cider vinegar
- 1 tbsp dried mint
- 1 tbsp olive oil
- 1 teaspn mustard
- ¼ teaspn salt
- ¼ cup water

Directions:

1. Chop the beef roughly and sprinkle it with the apple cider vinegar, dried mint, mustard, olive oil, and salt.
2. Stir the meat and let it sit for 20 min to marinate.
3. Transfer the meat to the slow cooker and add water.
4. Cook the beef for 3 h on High.
5. When the beef is cooked, let it rest for 10 min and serve!

Nutrition: calories: 187, fat: 8.8, fiber: 0.2, carbs: 2.6, protein: 23.2

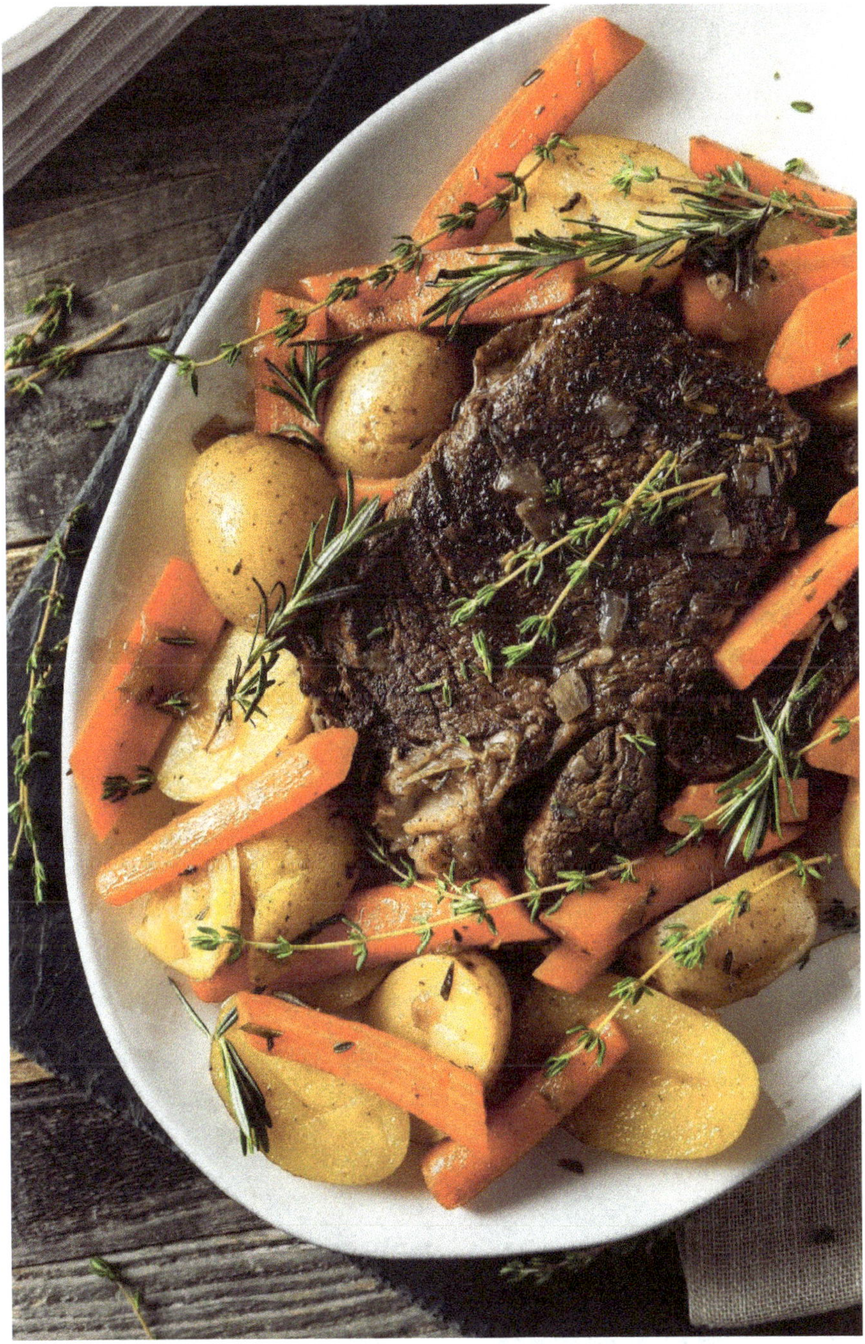

Chapter 4: Poultry

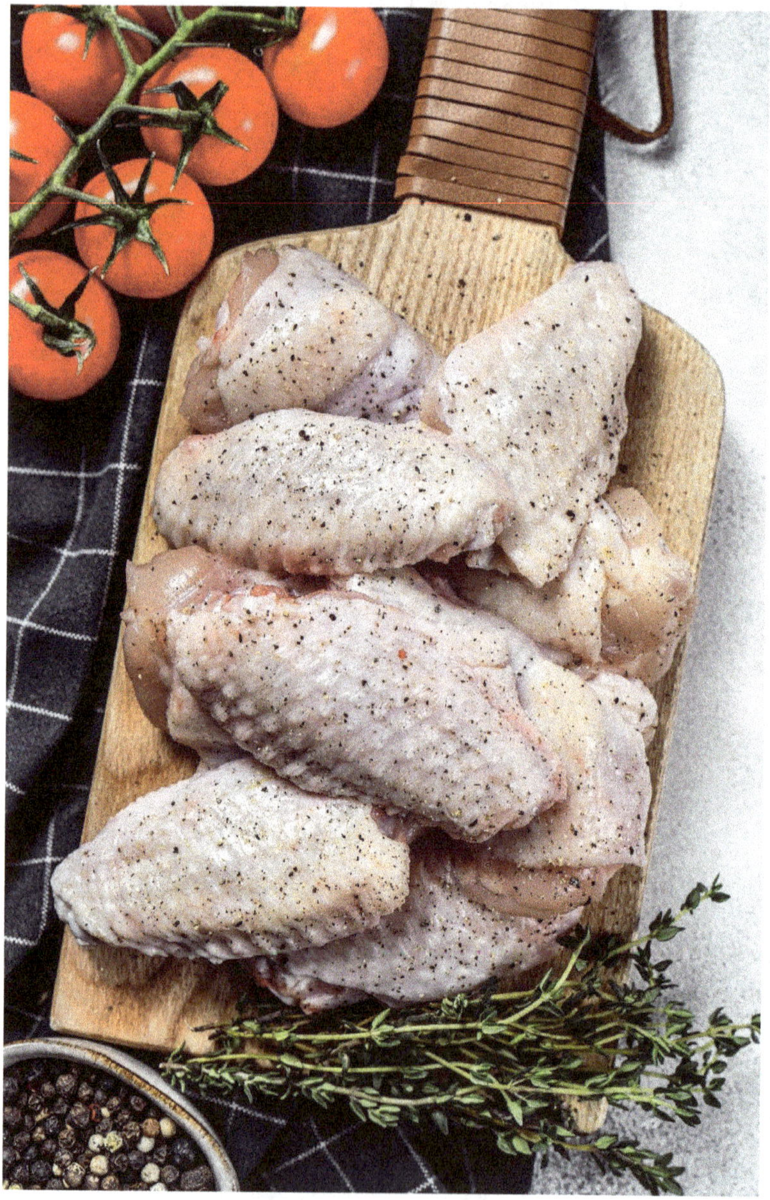

Green Peas Chowder

Preparation: 10 min | Cooking: 8 h | Servings: 6

Ingredients:

- 1-pound chicken breast, skinless, boneless, chopped
- 2 cups water
- 1 cup green peas
- ¼ cup Greek Yogurt
- 1 tbsp dried basil
- 1 teaspn ground black pepper
- ½ teaspn salt

Directions

1. Mix salt, chicken breast, ground black pepper, and dried basil.
2. Transfer the ingredients to the slow cooker.
3. Add water, green peas, yogurt, and close the lid.
4. Cook the chowder on Low for 8 h.

Duck Breast

Preparation: 10 min | Cooking: 5 h | Servings: 4

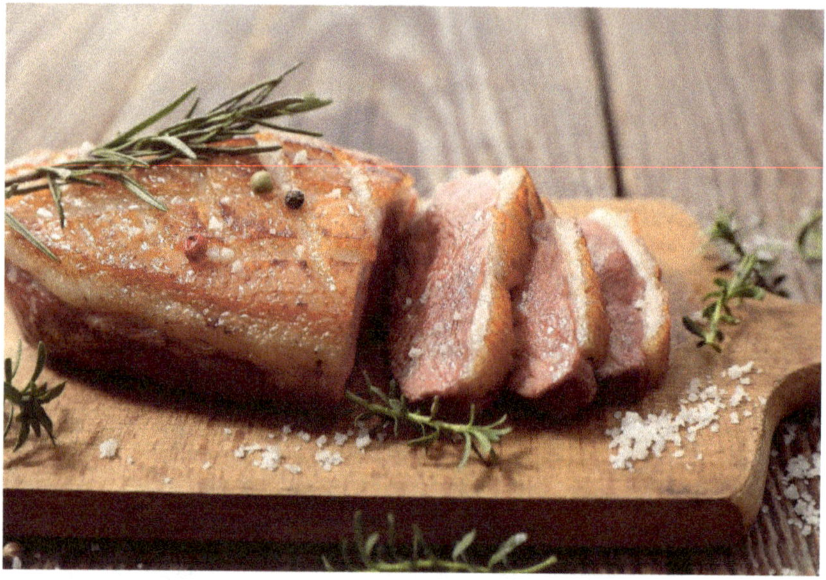

Ingredients:

- 1 teaspn liquid stevia
- 1-pound duck breast, boneless, skinless
- 1 teaspn chili pepper
- 2 tsps butter
- ½ cup water
- 1 bay leaf

Directions:

1. Rub the duck breast with the chili pepper and liquid stevia, then transfer it to the slow cooker.
2. Add the bay leaf and water.
3. Add butter and close the lid.
4. Cook the duck breast for 5 h on Low.
5. Let the cooked duck breast rest for 10 min, then remove it from the slow cooker.
6. Slice it into the servings.
7. Enjoy!

Nutrition: calories 199 Fat: 10.3, Fiber: 0.1, Carbs: 0.3, Protein: 25.1

Sugar Chicken

Preparation: 10 min | Cooking: 6 h | Servings: 6

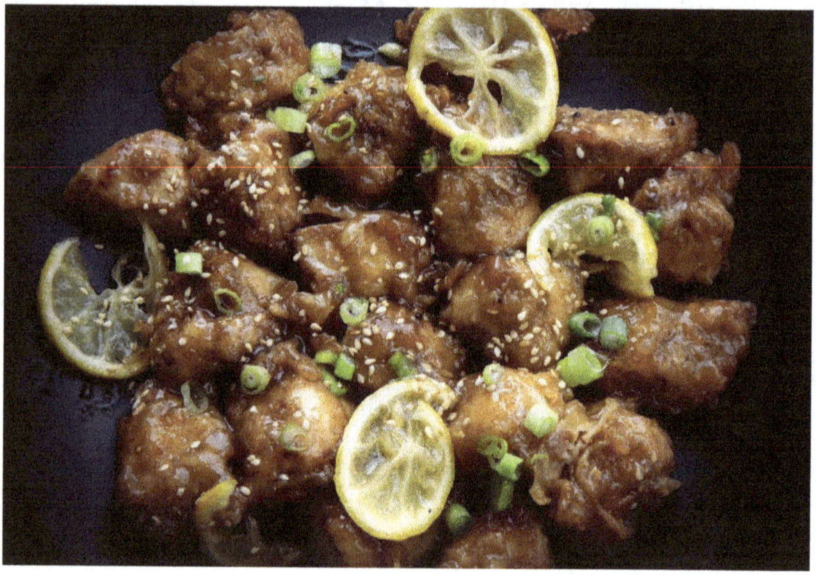

Ingredients:

- 1 teaspn chili flakes
- chicken drumsticks
- 1 tsps brown sugar
- 1 tbsp butter, melted
- 1 tbsp lemon juice
- 1 teaspn ground black pepper
- ¼ cup milk

Directions

1. In the bowl, mix chili flakes, brown sugar, butter, lemon juice, and ground black pepper.
2. Then brush every chicken drumstick with the sweet mixture and transfer to the slow cooker.
3. Add milk and close the lid. Cook the meal on Low for 6 h.

Basil Chicken

Preparation: 15 min | Cooking: 7 h | Servings: 4

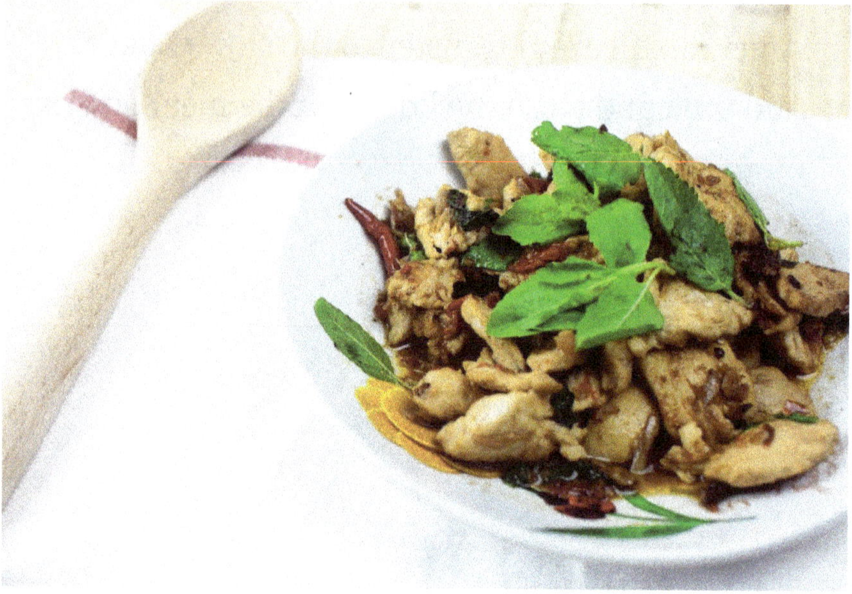

Ingredients:

- 2 tsps balsamic vinegar
- 1 cup of water
- 1 teaspn dried basil
- 1 teaspn dried oregano
- 1-pound chicken fillet, sliced
- 1 teaspn mustard

Directions:

1. Mix chicken fillet with mustard and balsamic vinegar.
2. Add dried basil, oregano, and transfer to the slow cooker.
3. Add water and close the lid.
4. Cook the chicken on low for 7 h.

Sweet Chicken Breast

Preparation: 20 min | Cooking: 4 h | Servings: 4

Ingredients:

- 2 red onions
- 2 tsps of liquid honey
- 1 tbsp butter
- ½ cup of water
- 1-pound chicken breast, skinless, boneless
- 1 teaspn curry paste

Directions:

1. Rub the chicken breast with curry paste and transfer to the slow cooker.
2. Slice the onion and add it to the cooker too.
3. Then add water and close the lid.
4. Cook the chicken breast on High for 4 h.
5. After this, toss the butter in the skillet.
6. Melt it and add chicken.
7. Sprinkle the chicken with liquid honey and roast for 1 minute per side.
8. Slice the chicken breast.

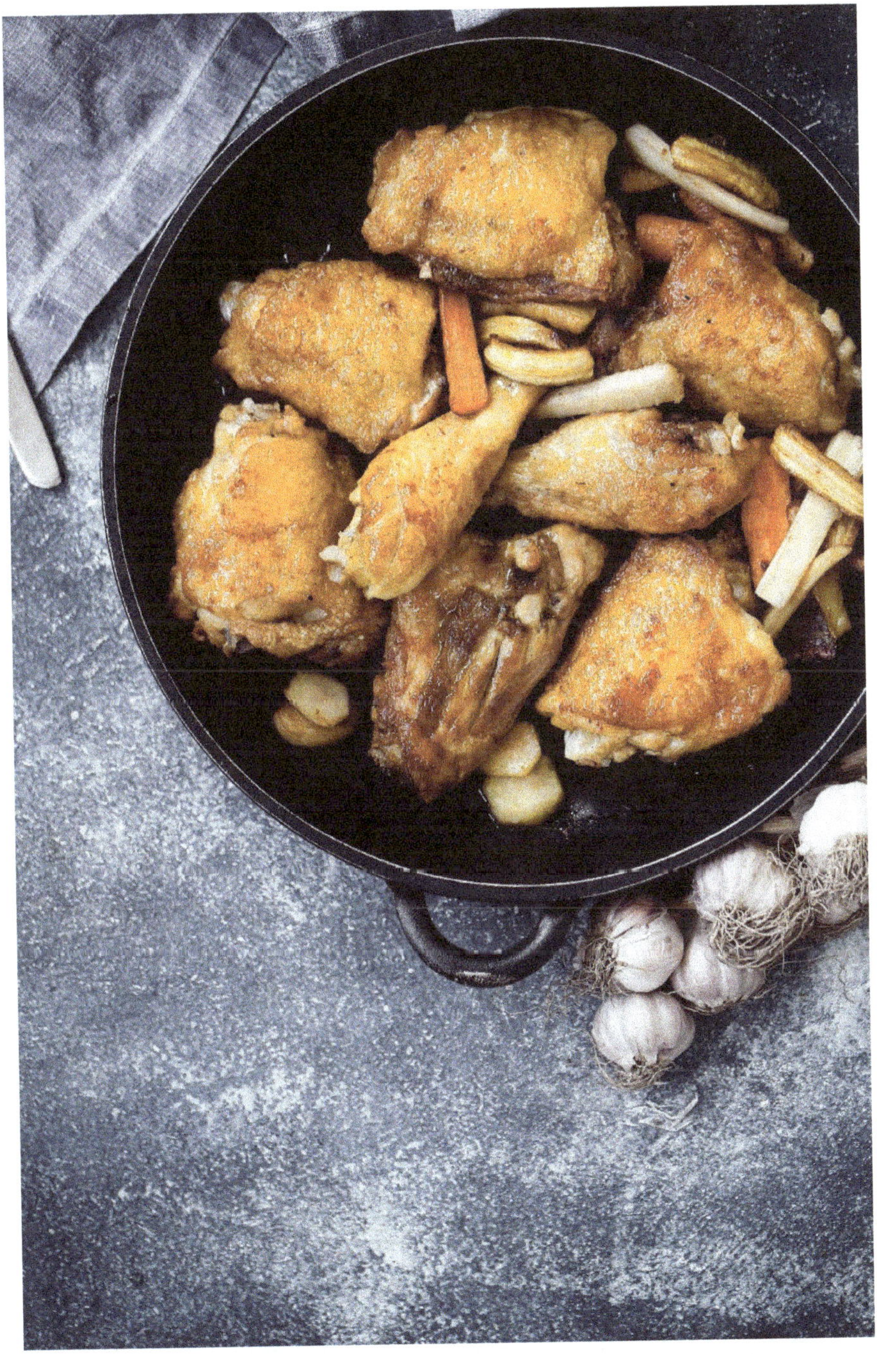

Chapter 5: Fish and Seafood

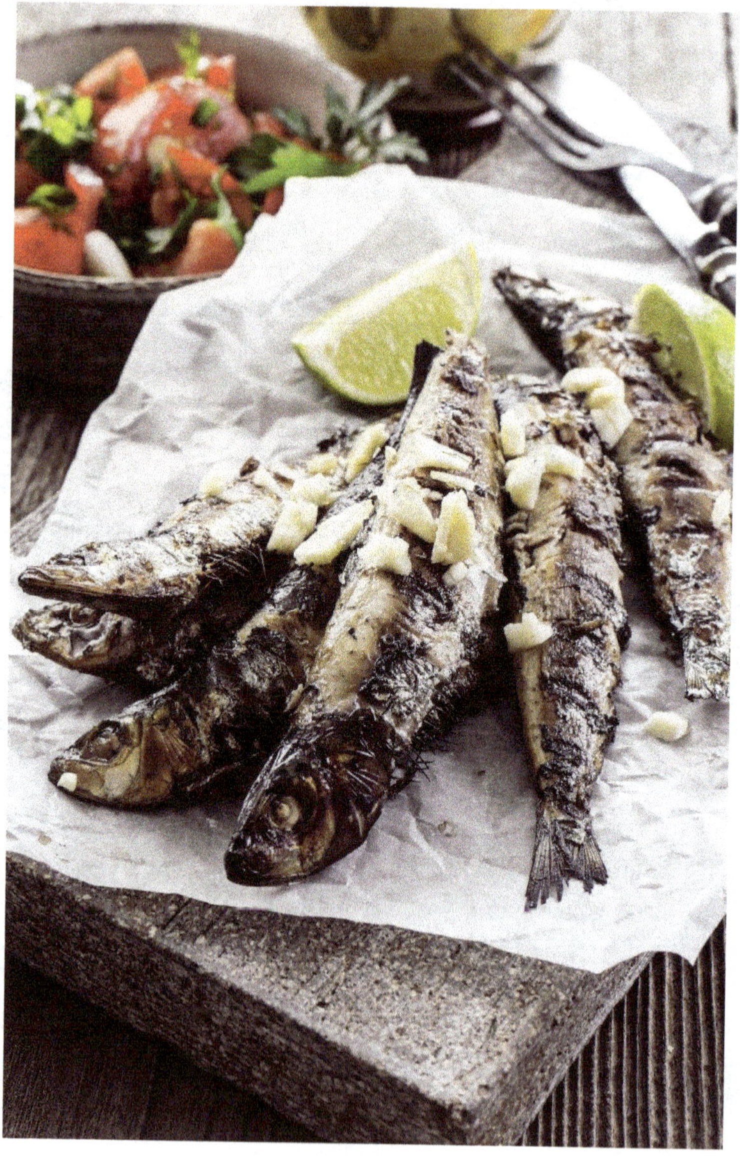

Chili Prawns

Servings: 6 | Preparation: 5 min | Cooking: 1 hour and 25 min

Ingredients:

- 18-ounce wild-caught prawns, shell-on
- ½ cup sliced scallions
- 1 thumb-sized ginger, minced
- 1 bulb of garlic, peeled and minced
- 1 tbsp swerve sweetener
- 2 tsps apple cider vinegar
- 2 tsps Sambal Oelek
- 1 tbsp fish sauce, unsweetened
- 4 tsps sesame oil
- ½ cup tomato ketchup, keto and unsweetened
- 1 egg, beaten

Directions:

1. Place all the ingredients, except for prawns, oil, and egg in a 6-quart slow cooker and stir until mixed.
2. Plug in the slow cooker, shut with lid and cook for 1 hour at high heat setting.

3. Then add prawns and continue cooking for 15 min at high heat setting or until prawns turn pink.
4. Stir in oil and egg and cook for 10 min.
5. Drizzle with more fish sauce and serve.

Nutrition: Net Carbs: 3.1g; Calories: 163.3; Total Fat: 10.7g; Saturated Fat: 1.8g; Protein: 13g; Carbs: 3.6g; Fiber: 0.5g; Sugar: 1.7g Total Fat: 59%; Protein: 32%; Carbs: 9%;

Lemon Pepper Tilapia

Servings: 6 | Preparation: 5 min | Cooking: 3 hours

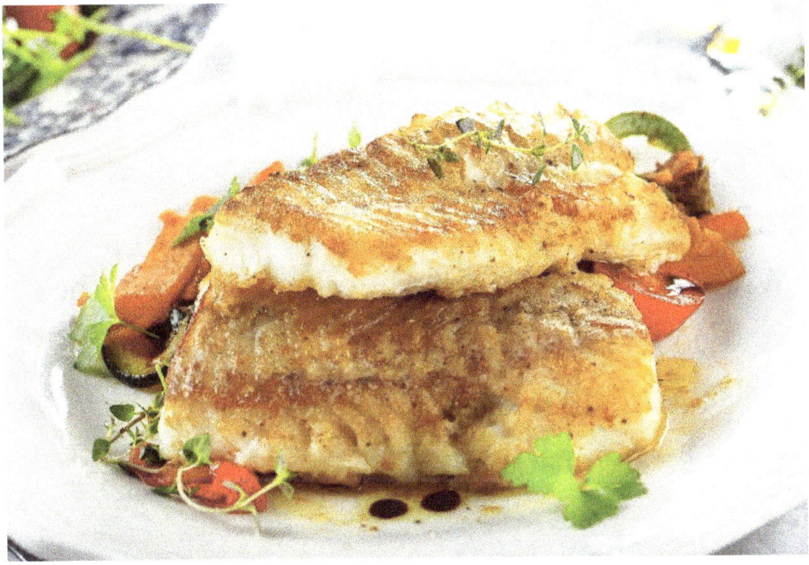

Ingredients:

- 6 wild-caught Tilapia fillets
- 4 teaspns lemon-pepper seasoning, divided
- 6 tsps unsalted butter, divided
- 1|2 cup lemon juice, fresh

Directions:

1. Cut a large piece of aluminum foil for each fillet and then arrange them on a clean working space.

2. Place each fillet in the middle of the foil, then season with lemon-pepper seasoning, drizzle with lemon juice and top with 1 tbsp butter.
3. Gently crimp the edges of foil to form a packet and place it into a 6-quart slow cooker.
4. Plug in the slow cooker, shut with lid and cook for 3 hours at high heat setting or until cooked through.
5. When done, carefully remove packets from the slow cooker and open the crimped edges and check the fish, it should be tender and flaky.
6. Serve straightaway.

Nutrition: Net Carbs: 1.2 g; Calories: 201.2; Total Fat: 12.9g; Saturated Fat: 9.1g; Protein: 19.6g; Carbs: 1.5g; Fiber: 0.3g; Sugar: 0.7g Total Fat: 58%; Protein: 39%; Carbs: 3%;

Vietnamese Braised Catfish

Servings: 3 | Preparation: 5 min | Cooking: 6 hours

Ingredients:

- 1 fillet of wild-caught catfish, cut into bite-size pieces
- 1 scallion, chopped
- 3 red chilies, chopped
- 1 tbsp grated ginger
- 1|2 cup swerve sweetener
- 2 tsps avocado oil
- 1|4 cup fish sauce, unsweetened

Directions:

1. Place a small saucepan over medium heat, add sweetener and cook until it melts.
2. Then add scallion, chilies, ginger and fish sauce and stir until mixed.
3. Transfer this mixture in a 4-quart slow cooker, add fish and toss until coated.
4. Plug in the slow cooker, shut with lid and cook for 6 hours at low heat setting until cooked.
5. Drizzle with avocado oil and serve straightaway.

Nutrition: Net Carbs: 0.1g; Calories: 110.7; Total Fat: 8g; Saturated Fat: 1.2g; Protein: 9.4g; Carbs: 0.3g; Fiber: 0.2g; Sugar: 0.2g Total Fat: 65%; Protein: 34%; Carbs: 1%;

Lemon Dill Halibut

Servings: 2 | Preparation: 5 min | Cooking: 2 hours

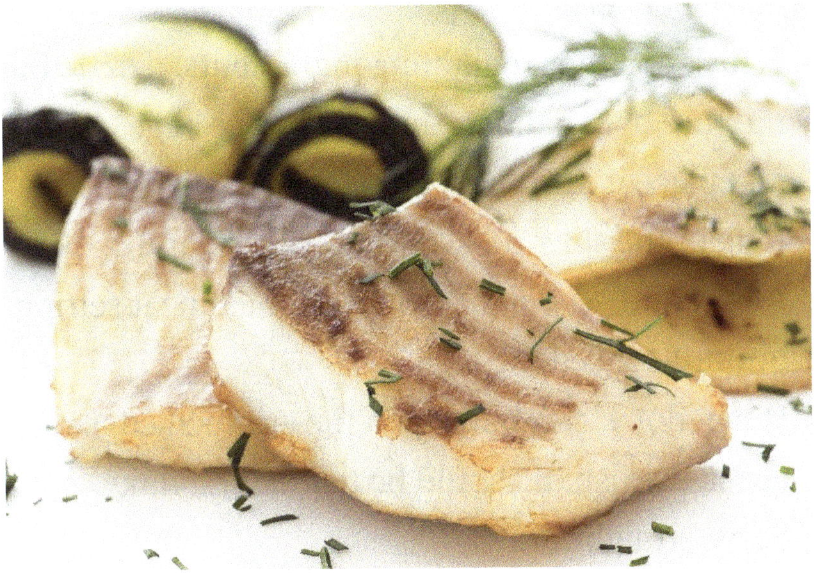

Ingredients:

- 12-ounce wild-caught halibut fillet
- 1 teaspn salt
- ½ teaspn ground black pepper
- 1 1/2 teaspn dried dill
- 1 tbsp fresh lemon juice
- 3 tsps avocado oil

Directions:

1. Cut an 18-inch piece of aluminum foil, halibut fillet in the middle and then season with salt and black pepper.
2. Whisk together remaining ingredients, drizzle this mixture over halibut, then crimp the edges of foil and place it into a 6-quart slow cooker.
3. Plug in the slow cooker, shut with lid and cook for 1 hour and 30 min or 2 hours at high heat setting or until cooked through.
4. When done, carefully open the crimped edges and check the fish, it should be tender and flaky.
5. Serve straightaway.

Nutrition: Net Carbs: 0g; Calories: 321.5; Total Fat: 21.4g; Saturated Fat: 7.2g; Protein: 32.1g; Carbs: 0g; Fiber: 0g; Sugar: 0.6g Total Fat: 60%; Protein: 40%; Carbs: 0%;

Clam Chowder

Servings: 6 | Preparation: 5 min | Cooking: 6 hours

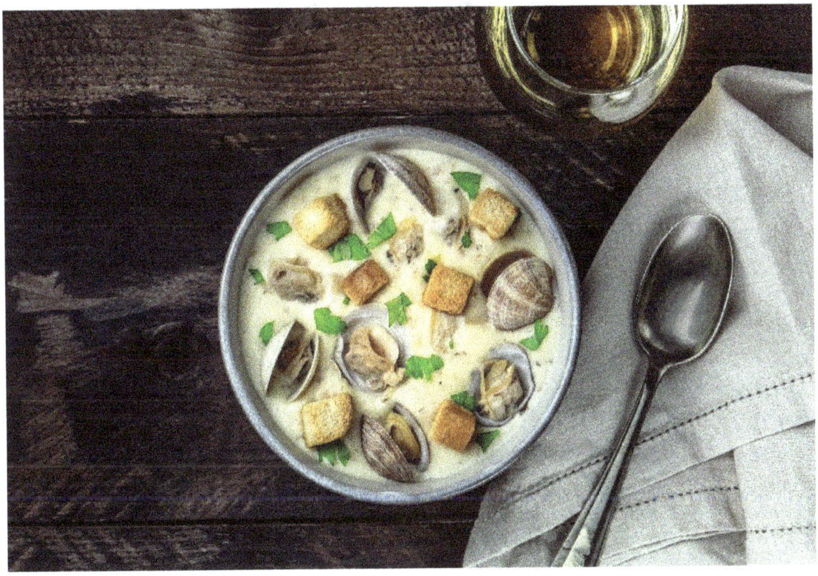

Ingredients:

- 20-ounce wild-caught baby clams, with juice
- ½ cup chopped scallion
- ½ cup chopped celery
- 1 teaspn salt
- 1 teaspn ground black pepper
- 1 teaspn dried thyme
- 1 tbsp avocado oil
- 2 cups coconut cream, full-fat

- 2 cups chicken broth

Directions:

1. Grease a 6-quart slow cooker with oil, add ingredients and stir until mixed.
2. Plug in the slow cooker, shut with lid and cook for 4 to 6 hours at low heat setting or until cooked through.
3. Serve straightaway.

Nutrition: Net Carbs: 6.8g; Calories: 357; Total Fat: 28.9g; Saturated Fat: 13.2g; Protein: 15.2g; Carbs: 8.9g; Fiber: 2.1g; Sugar: 3.9g Total Fat: 73%; Protein: 17%; Carbs: 10%;

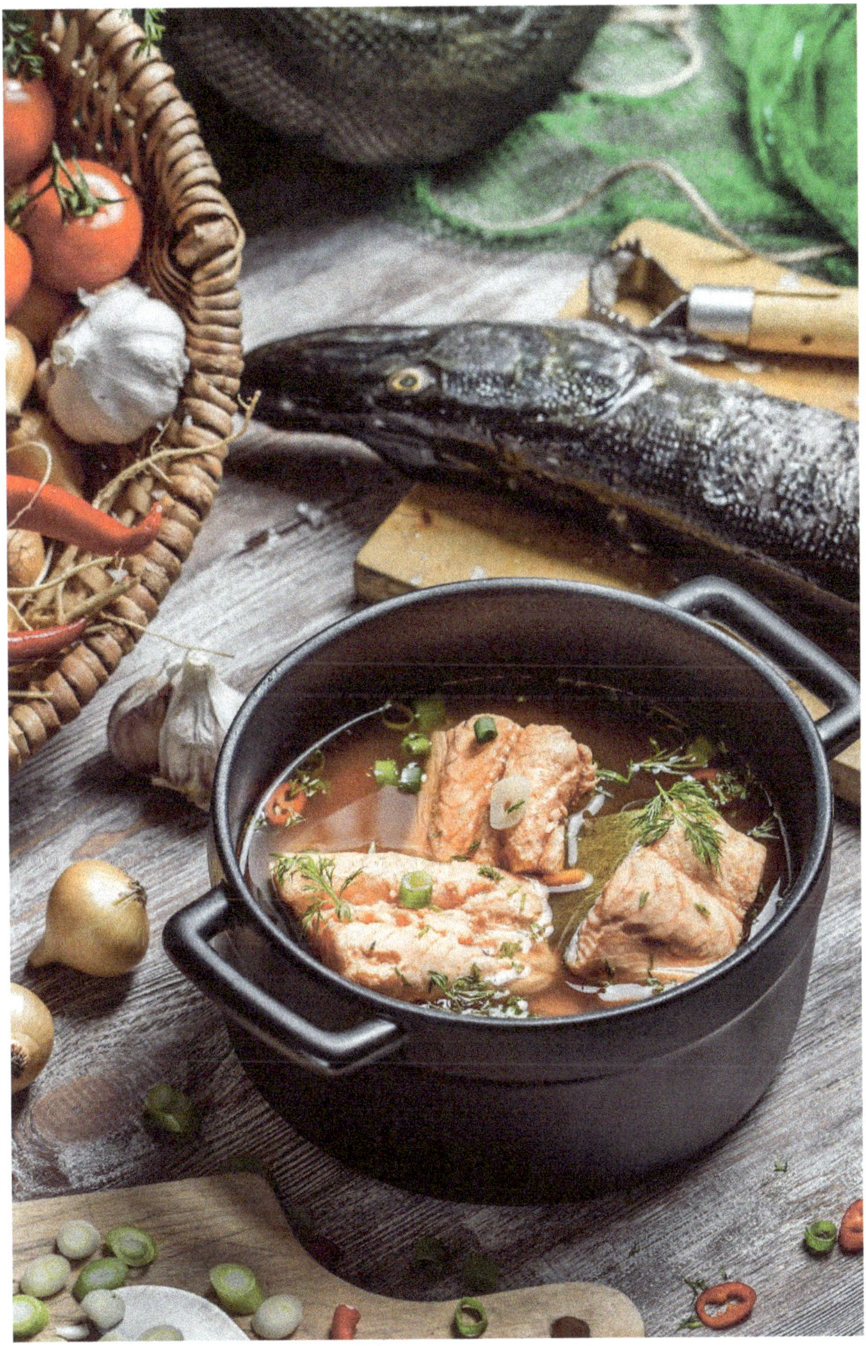

Chapter 6: Vegetable Meals

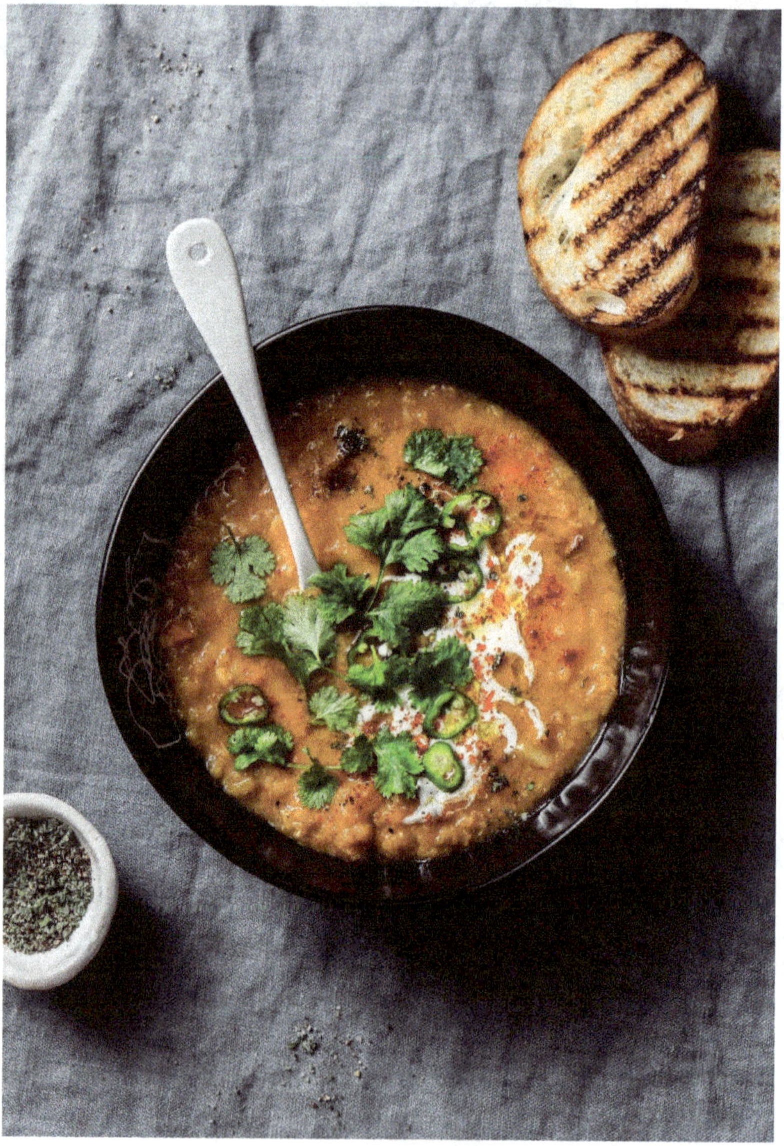

Mashed Turnips

Preparation: 10 min | Cooking: 7 h | Servings: 6

Ingredients

- 3-pounds turnip, chopped
- 2 cup water
- 1 tbsp vegan butter
- 1 tbsp chives, chopped
- oz. Parmesan, grated

Directions

1. Put turnips in the slow cooker.
2. Add water and cook the vegetables on low for 7 h.
3. Then drain water and mash the turnips.
4. Add chives, butter, and Parmesan.
5. Carefully stir the mixture until butter and Parmesan are melted.
6. Then add chives. Mix the mashed turnips again.

Sautéed Greens

Preparation: 15 min | Cooking: 1 hour | Servings: 4

Ingredients

- 1 cup spinach, chopped
- 2 cups collard greens, chopped
- 1 cup Swiss chard, chopped
- water
- ½ cup half and half

Directions

1. Put spinach, collard greens, and Swiss chard in the slow cooker.
2. Add water and close the lid.
3. Cook the greens on High for 1 hour.
4. Then drain water and transfer the greens in the bowl.
5. Bring the half and half to boil and pour over greens.
6. Carefully mix the greens.

Potato Salad

Preparation: 10 min | Cooking: 3 h | Servings: 2

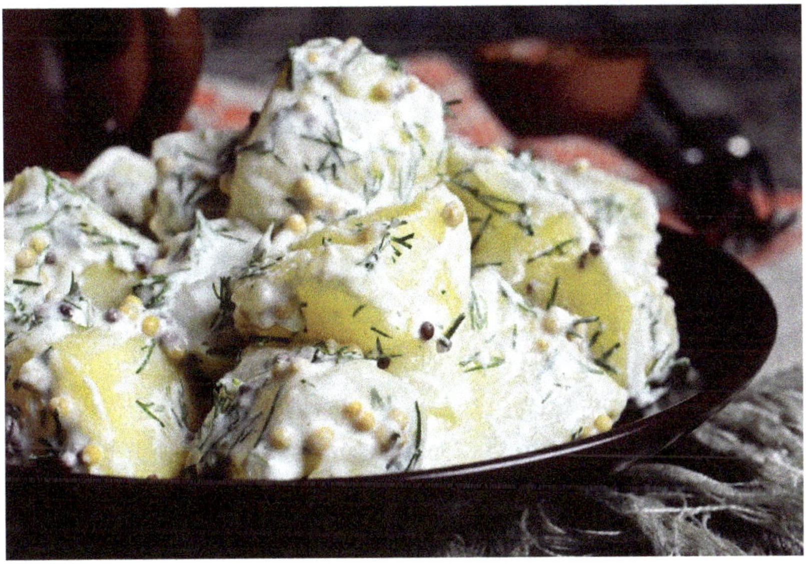

Ingredients

- 1 cup potato, chopped
- 1 cup of water
- 1 teaspn salt
- oz. celery stalk, chopped
- oz. fresh parsley, chopped
- ¼ onion, diced
- 1 tbsp mayonnaise

Directions

1. Put the potatoes in the slow cooker.
2. Add water and salt.
3. Cook the potatoes on High for 3 h.
4. Then drain water and transfer the potatoes in the salad bowl.
5. Add all remaining ingredients and carefully mix the salad.

Spicy Pecans

Preparation: 10 min | Cooking: 3 h | Servings: 16

Ingredients

- lbs. pecan halves
- tbsp. Cajun seasoning blend
- tbsp. olive oil

Directions

1. Add all ingredients to the slow cooker and stir well to combine.
2. Cover slow cooker with lid and cook on low for 1 hour.
3. Stir well. Cover again and cook for 2 h more.
4. Serve and enjoy.

Nutrition: Calories: 607 Fat: 62.5 g Carbohydrates 12.2 g Sugar 3 g Protein: 9.1 g Cholesterol 0 mg

Ranch Broccoli

Preparation: 10 min | Cooking: 1.5 h | Servings: 3

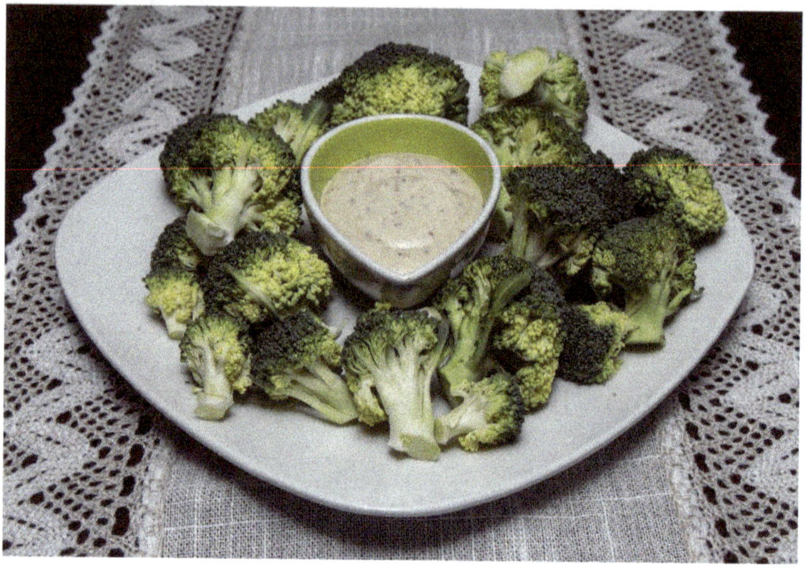

Ingredients

- 2 cups broccoli
- 1 teaspn chili flakes
- 2 tsps ranch dressing
- 2 cups of water

Directions

1. Put the broccoli in the slow cooker.
2. Add water and close the lid.

3. Cook the broccoli on high for 1.5 h.
4. Then drain water and transfer the broccoli in the bowl.
5. Sprinkle it with chili flakes and ranch dressing. Shake the meal gently.

Chapter 7: Side Dishes

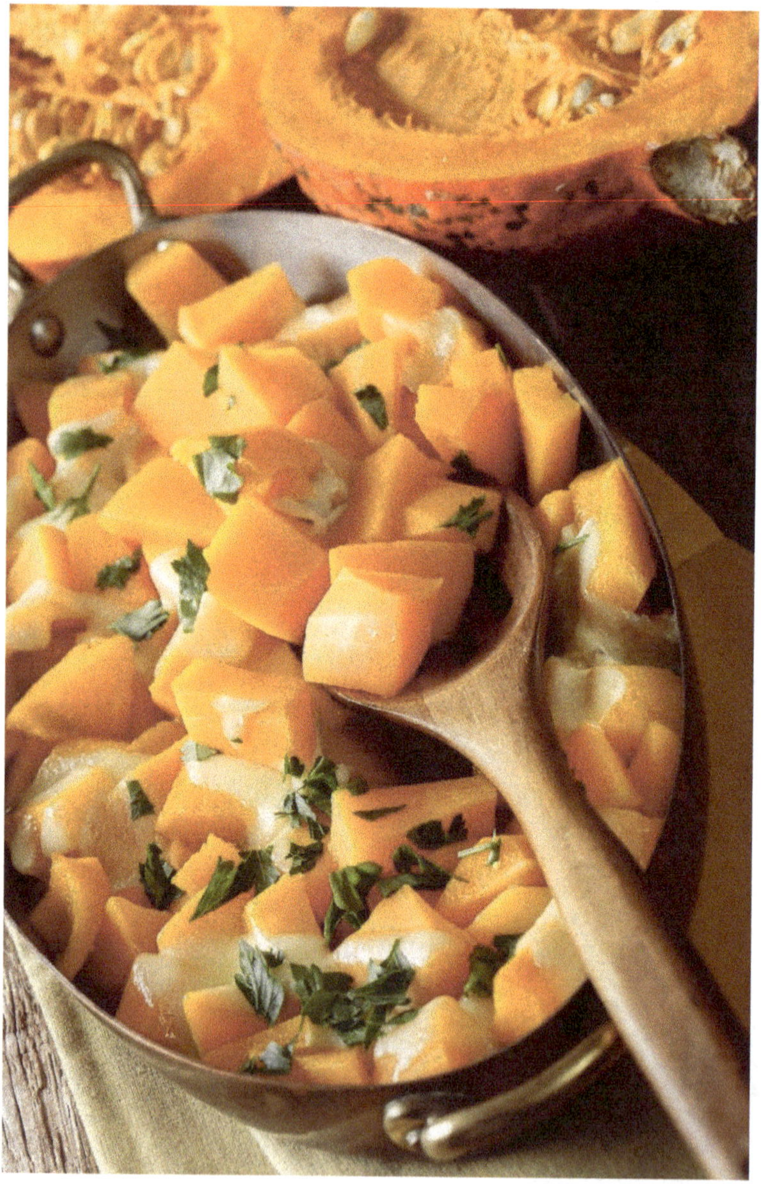

Soy-Ginger Steamed Pompano

Servings: 4 | Preparation: 5 min | Cooking: 1 hour

Ingredients

- 1 wild-caught whole pompano, gutted and scaled
- 1 bunch scallion, diced
- 1 bunch cilantro, chopped
- 3 teaspns minced garlic
- 1 tbsp grated ginger
- 1 tbsp swerve sweetener
- ¼ cup soy sauce
- ¼ cup white wine
- ¼ cup sesame oil

Directions

1. Place scallions in a 6-quart slow cooker and top with fish.
2. Whisk together remaining ingredients, except for cilantro, and pour the mixture all over the fish.
3. Plug in the slow cooker, shut with lid and cook for 1 hour at high heat setting or until cooked through.
4. Garnish with cilantro and serve.

Nutrition: Net Carbs: 3.5g; Calories: 202.5; Total Fat: 24.2g; Saturated Fat: 6g; Protein: 22.7g; Carbs: 4g; Fiber: 0.5g; Sugar: 1.1g Total Fat: 67%; Protein: 28%; Carbs: 5%;

Seabass in Coconut Cream Sauce

Servings: 3 | Preparation: 5 min | Cooking: 1 hour and 30 min

Ingredients

- 18-ounce wild-caught sea bass
- 5 jalapeno peppers
- 4 stalks of bok choy
- 2 stalks of scallions, sliced
- 1 tbsp grated ginger
- 1 ½ teaspn salt
- 1 tbsp fish sauce, unsweetened
- 2 cups coconut cream

Directions

1. Stir all the ingredients except for bok choy and fish in a bowl and add this mixture in a 6-quarts slow cooker.
2. Plug in the slow cooker, then add fish, top with bok choy and shut with lid.
3. Cook sea bass for 1 hour and 30 min or until cooked.
4. Serve straightaway.

Nutrition: Net Carbs: 5.9g; Calories: 760; Total Fat: 56.5g; Saturated Fat: 40.4g; Protein: 49.4g; Carbs: 13.3g; Fiber: 7.4g; Sugar: 8g Total Fat: 67%; Protein: 26%; Carbs: 7%;

Mahi Mahi Taco Wraps

Servings: 6 | Preparation: 5 min | Cooking: 2 hours

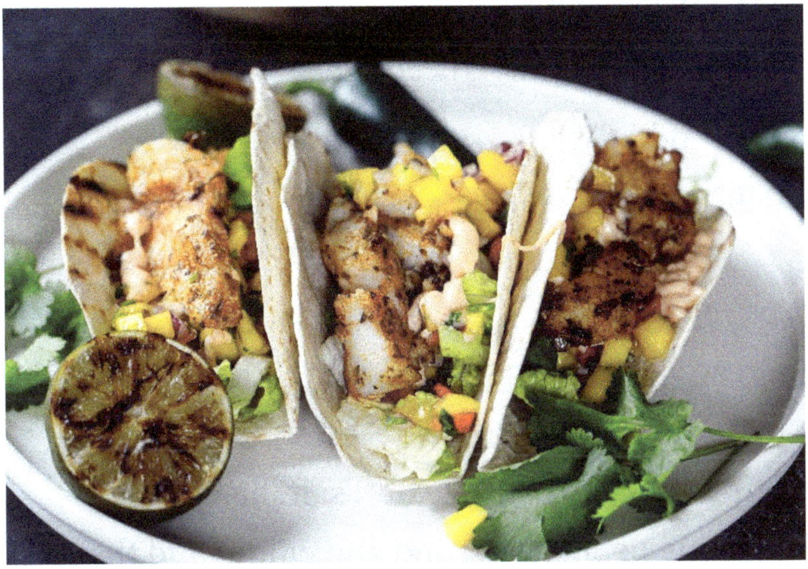

Ingredients

- 1 pound Mahi Mahi, wild-caught
- ½ cup cherry tomatoes
- 1 small green bell pepper, cored and sliced
- 1|4 of a medium red onion, thinly sliced
- ½ teaspn garlic powder
- 1 teaspn sea salt
- ½ teaspn ground black pepper
- 1 teaspn chipotle pepper

- ½ teaspn dried oregano
- 1 teaspn cumin
- 2 tsps avocado oil
- 1|4 cup chicken stock
- 1 medium avocado, diced
- 1 cup sour cream
- 6 large lettuce leaves

Directions

1. Grease a 6-quarts slow cooker with oil, place fish in it and then pour in chicken stock.
2. Stir together garlic powder, salt, black pepper, chipotle pepper, oregano and cumin and then season fish with half of this mixture.
3. Layer fish with tomatoes, pepper and onion, season with remaining spice mixture and shut with lid.
4. Plug in the slow cooker and cook fish for 2 hours at high heat setting or until cooked through.
5. When done, evenly spoon fish among lettuce, top with avocado and sour cream and serve.

Nutrition: Net Carbs: 2g; Calories: 193.6; Total Fat: 12g; Saturated Fat: 1.7g; Protein: 17g; Carbs: 5g;

Fiber: 3g; Sugar: 2.5g Total Fat: 55%; Protein: 35%; Carbs: 10%;

Beef and Cheese Stuffed Tomatoes

Servings: 4 | Preparation: 5 min | Cooking: 4 hours

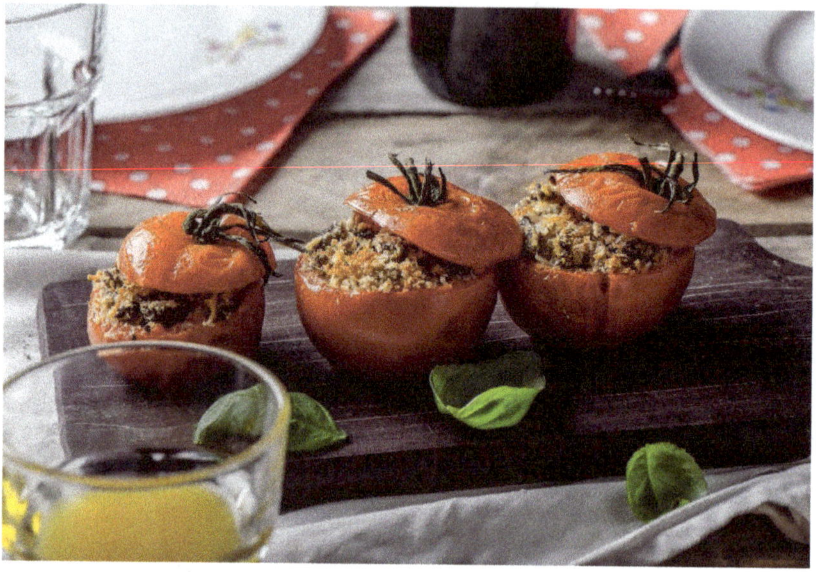

Ingredients

- ¼ pound ground beef, grass-fed
- 4 large tomatoes
- 1 green pepper, chopped
- 1 stalk of green onion, chopped
- ½ teaspn salt
- ½ teaspn ground black
- ½ teaspn dried parsley
- 4 tsps avocado oil

- ¾ cup beef broth
- 6 tsps grated Mozzarella cheese
- 6 tbsp grated parmesan cheese

Directions

1. Remove top off from each tomato and then scoop out its pulp with a small spoon.
2. Transfer tomato pulp into a large bowl, add beef, green pepper, onion, salt, and black pepper and stir until combined.
3. Spoon this mixture into each tomato, then sprinkle 1 ½ tbsp of mozzarella and parmesan cheese on top of each tomato, sprinkle with parsley and then brush with oil.
4. Plug in 4-quarts slow cooker, then pour in beef broth, add stuffed tomatoes and shut with lid.
5. Cook for 2 to 4 hours at high heat setting or until tomatoes are tender.
6. Serve straightaway.

Nutrition: Net Carbs: 6.5g; Calories: 369; Total Fat: 30.3g; Saturated Fat: 17g; Protein: 15g; Carbs: 9.2g; Fiber: 3.3g; Sugar: 6g Total Fat: 74%; Protein: 16%; Carbs: 10%;

Reuben Soup

Servings: 12 | Preparation: 5 min | Cooking: 7 hours

Ingredients

- 2 pounds grass-fed corned beef, diced
- 1 pound sauerkraut
- 1 medium white onion, peeled and diced
- 1 ½ teaspn minced garlic
- 1 teaspn coriander seeds
- 1 teaspn dill seeds
- 1/2 teaspn celery seeds
- 1 tbsp mustard seeds
- 2 tsps unsalted butter
- 8 cups beef broth
- 2 cups heavy cream
- 8 ounce shredded Swiss cheese

Directions

1. Place a medium skillet pan over medium heat, add 1 tbsp butter and when it melts, add onion and cook for 5 min or until tender.
2. Then add garlic and continue cooking for 1 minute or until fragrant.

3. Spoon this mixture into a 6-quart slow cooker, along with remaining ingredients except for cream and cheese and stir until mixed.
4. Plug in the slow cooker, then shut with lid and cook for 7 hours at low heat setting or 3 ½ hours at high heat setting.
5. When 1 hour of the cooking hour is left, stir in cream and cheese and continue cooking until cooked through.
6. Serve straightaway.

Nutrition: Net Carbs: 1.9g; Calories: 343; Total Fat: 26.3g; Saturated Fat: 11g; Protein: 23g; Carbs: 3.4g; Fiber: 1.5g; Sugar: 5g Total Fat: 69%; Protein: 27%; Carbs: 4%;

Chapter 8: Snack and Appetizers

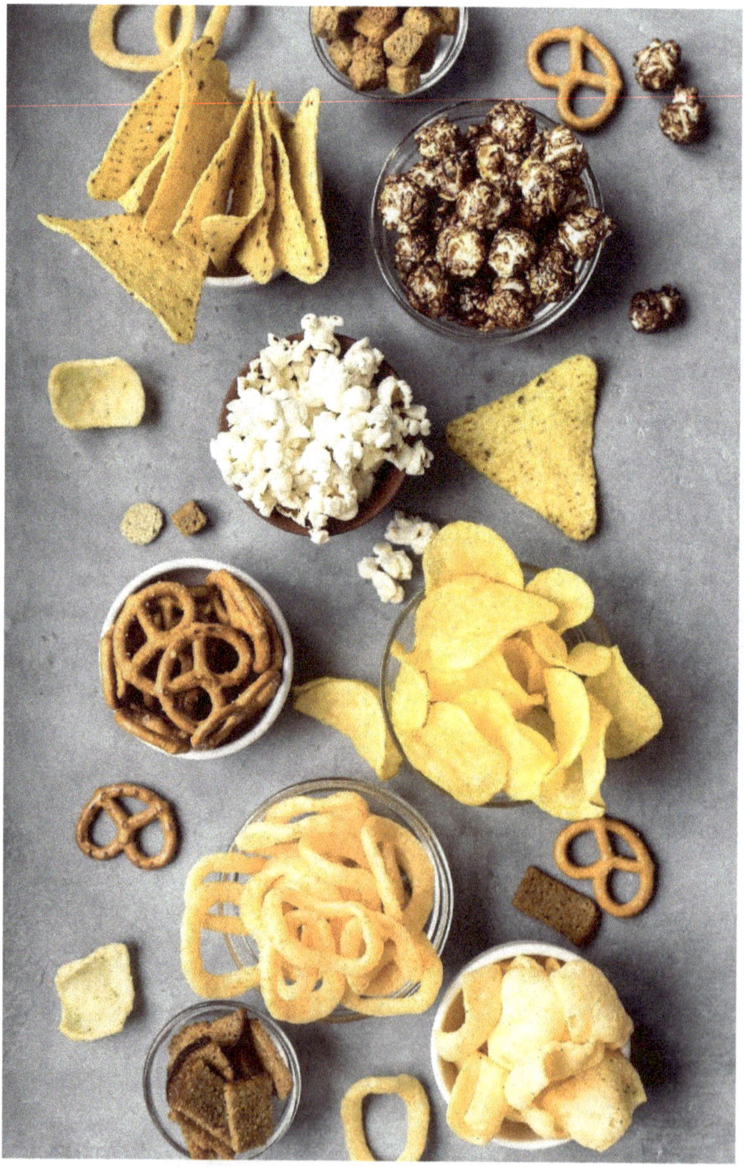

Stuffed Jalapenos

Preparation: 10 min | Cooking: 4.5 h | Servings: 3

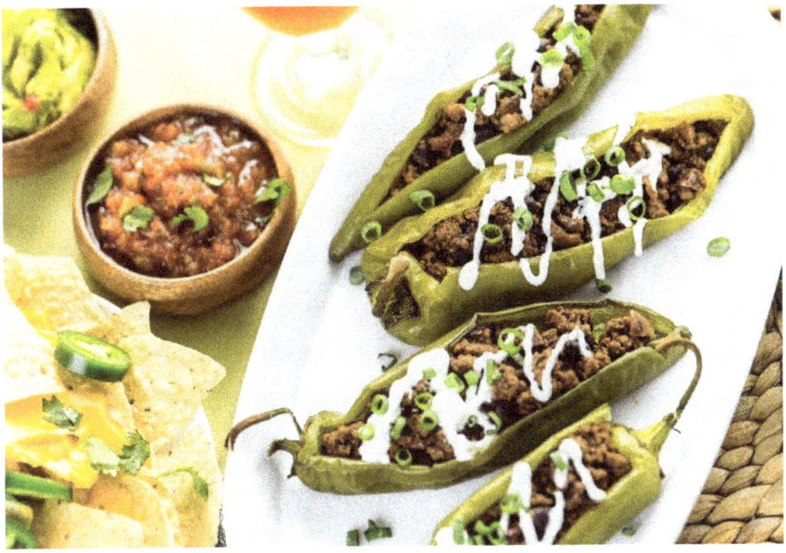

Ingredients

- jalapenos, deseed
- oz. minced beef
- 1 teaspn garlic powder
- ½ cup of water

Directions

1. Mix the minced beef with garlic powder.
2. Then fill the jalapenos with minced meat and arrange it in the slow cooker.

3. Add water and cook the jalapenos on High for 4.5 h.

Flavorful Mexican Cheese Dip

Preparation: 10 min | Cooking: 1 hour | Servings: 6

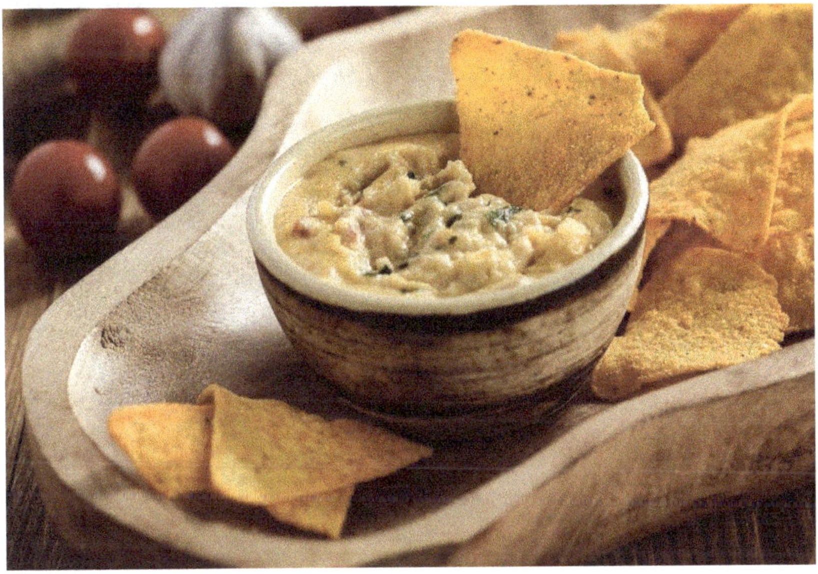

Ingredients

- 1 tsp taco seasoning
- ¾ cup tomatoes with green chilies
- oz. Velveeta cheese, cut into cube

Directions

1. Add cheese into the slow cooker. Cover and cook on low for 30 min. Stir occasionally.
2. Add taco seasoning and tomatoes with green chilies and stir well.

3. Cover again and cook on low for 30 min more.
4. Stir well and serve.

Nutrition: Calories: 159 Fat: 12.6 g Carbohydrates 1.9 g Sugar 0.3 g Protein: 9.6 g

Cheese Chicken Dip

Preparation: 10 min | Cooking: 2 h | Servings: 10

Ingredients

- ½ cup bell peppers, chopped
- 1 cup chicken breast, cooked and shredded
- oz. can tomato with green chilies
- ½ lb. cheese, cubed

Directions

1. Add all ingredients into the slow cooker and stir well to combine.
2. Cover slow cooker with lid and cook on low for 2 h.
3. Stir well and serve.

Nutrition: Calories: 120 Fat: 8 g Carbohydrates 2 g Sugar 0.4 g Protein: 10 g

Easy Texas Dip

Preparation: 10 min | Cooking: 6 h | Servings: 8

Ingredients

- 1 ½ cups Velveeta cheese, cubed
- cups fresh tomatoes, diced
- oz can green chilies, diced
- 1 large onion, chopped

Directions

1. Add all ingredients into the slow cooker and stir well to combine.
2. Cover slow cooker with lid and cook on low for 6 h.
3. Stir well and serve.

Nutrition: Calories: 104 Fat: 7.2 g Carbohydrates 4.4 g Sugar 2.1 g Protein: 6 g Cholesterol 22 mg

Tasty Seasoned Mixed Nuts

Preparation: 10 min | Cooking: 2 h | Servings: 20

Ingredients

- cups mixed nuts
- tbsp. curry powder
- tbsp. butter, melted
- Salt

Directions

1. 1 Add all ingredients into the slow cooker and stir well to combine.
2. 2 Cover slow cooker with lid and cook on high for a ½ hour. Stir again and cook for 30 min more.
3. 3 Cover again and cook on low for 1 hour more.
4. 4 Stir well and serve.

Nutrition: Calories: 375 Fat: 34.7 g Carbohydrates 12.8 g Sugar 2.5 g Protein: 9 g Cholesterol 6 mg

Chapter 9: Dessert

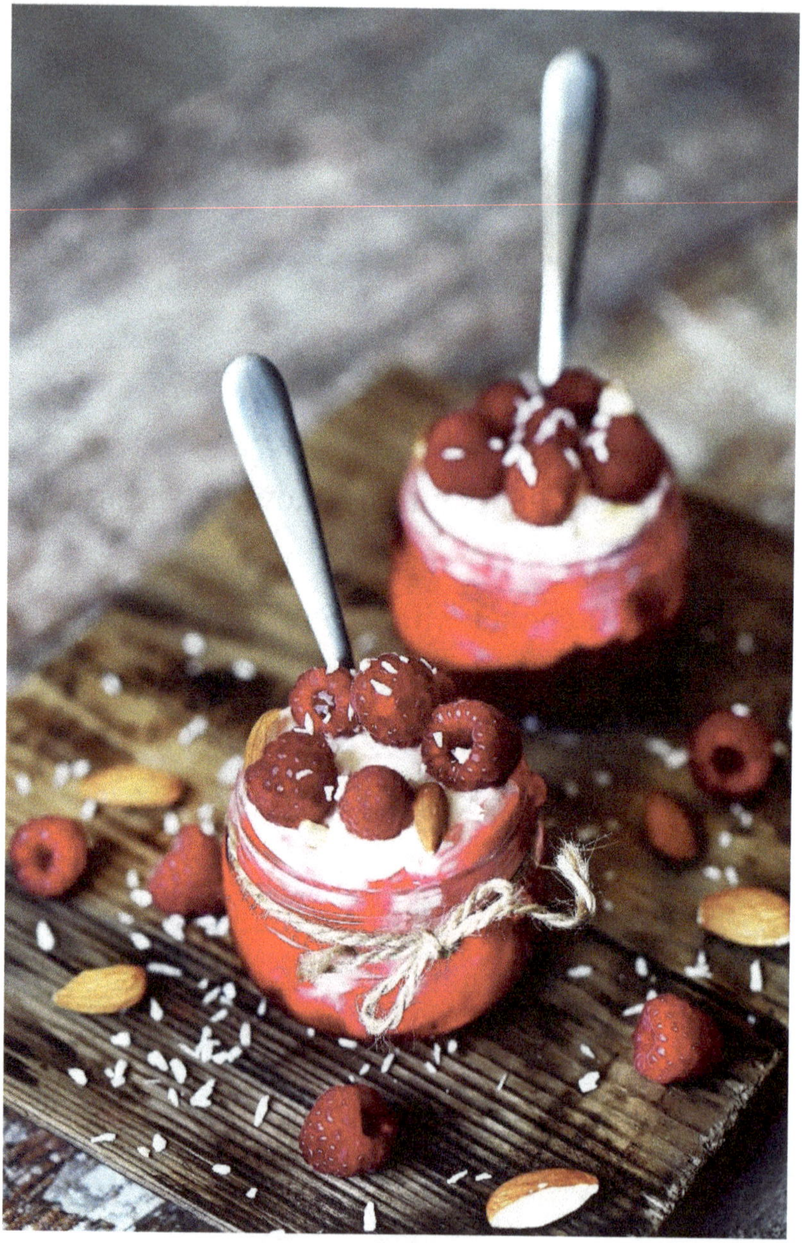

Chocolate Fudge

Preparation: 10 min | Cooking: 2 h | Servings: 30

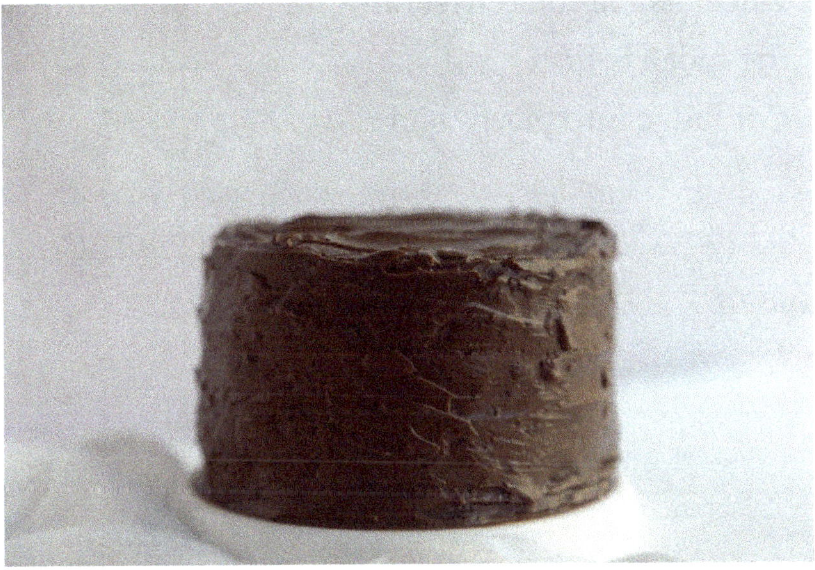

Ingredients

- ½ cups chocolate chips, sugar-free
- 1 tsp liquid stevia
- 1 tsp vanilla extract
- 1/3 cup unsweetened coconut milk

Directions

1. Add stevia, vanilla, chocolate chips, and coconut milk into the slow cooker and stir well.
2. Cover slow cooker with lid and cook on low for 2 h.

3. Open the lid and stir until smooth.
4. Grease casserole dish with butter and spread mixture into the dish.
5. Place dish in the refrigerator for 30 min or until the fudge is firm.
6. Cut fudge into pieces and serve.

Nutrition: Calories: 81 Fat: 4.8 g Carbohydrates 8.5 g Sugar 7.3 g Protein: 1.1 g Cholesterol 3 mg

Keto Cobbler

Preparation: 15 min | Cooking: 2 h | Servings: 4

Ingredients

- 1 cup blackberries
- 1 tbsp liquid stevia
- 1 teaspn Psyllium Husk
- 5 tsps almond flour
- 1 egg, beaten
- 1 tbsp butter

Directions

1. Whisk the egg and combine them with the almond flour and Psyllium Husk.
2. Add the liquid stevia and butter and knead into a smooth dough.
3. Chop the dough into small pieces.
4. Cover the bottom of the slow cooker with parchment.
5. Place a small amount of the dough in the bottom of the slow cooker.
6. Sprinkle the dough with a small amount of the blackberries.

7. Add a second layer of the chopped dough followed by more blackberries.
8. Continue layering until you use all the ingredients.
9. Close the lid and cook the cobbler for 2 h on High.
10. Let the cooked cobbler cool slightly.
11. Serve it!

Nutrition: calories: 264, fat: 21.7, fiber: 8, carbs: 13.9, protein: 9.4

Peanut Butter Oatmeal

Preparation: 10 min | Cooking: 8 h | Servings: 2

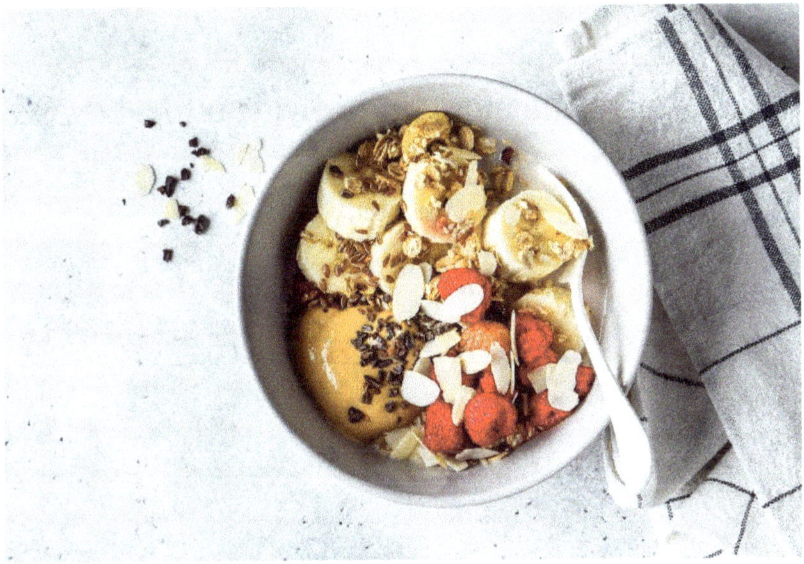

Ingredients

- 1 banana, mashed
- 1 and ½ cups almond milk
- ½ cup steel-cut oats
- 2 tsps peanut butter
- ½ teaspn vanilla extract
- ½ teaspn cinnamon powder
- ½ tbsp chia seeds

Directions

1. In your slow cooker, mix almond milk with banana, oats, peanut butter, vanilla extract, cinnamon, and chia, stir, cover, and cook on Low for 8 h.
2. Stir oatmeal one more time, divide into 2 bowls and serve.
3. Enjoy!

Nutrition: Calories: 222, Fat: 5, Fiber: 6, Carbs: 9, Protein: 11

Tomato Jam

Preparation: 10 min | Cooking: 3 h | Servings: 2

Ingredients

- ½ pound tomatoes, chopped
- 1 green apple, grated
- 2 tsps red wine vinegar
- 2 tsps sugar

Directions

1. In your slow cooker, mix the tomatoes with the apple with the other ingredients, put the lid on, and cook on Low for 3 h.
2. Whisk the jam well, blend a bit using an immersion blender, divide into bowls and serve cold.

Nutrition: Calories: 70, Fat: 1, Fiber: 1, Carbs: 18, Protein: 1

Applesauce

Preparation: 10 min | Cooking: 2 h | Servings: 6

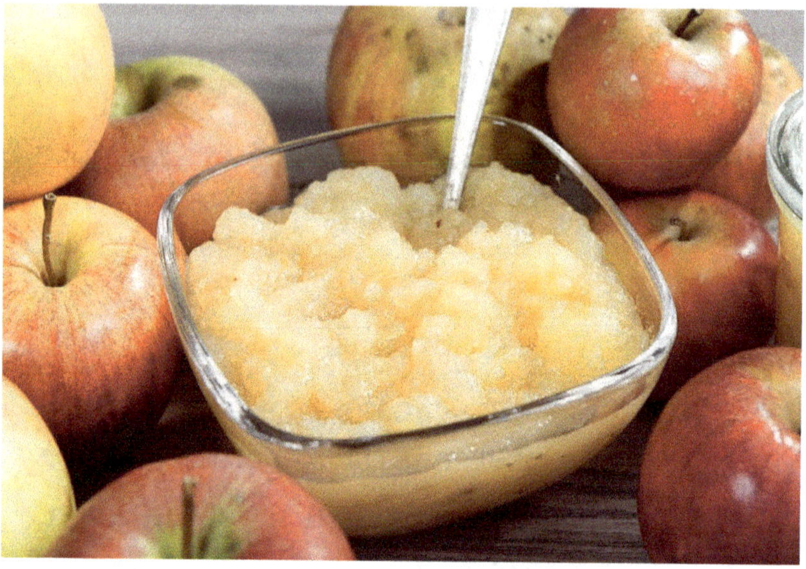

Ingredients

- lbs. fresh apples, peel, core, and slice
- 1/4 cup water
- whole cinnamon sticks
- 1 tbsp fresh lemon juice

Directions

1. Add all ingredients to the slow cooker and stir well.

2. Cover slow cooker with lid and cook on high for 2 h.
3. Discard cinnamon sticks and using a potato masher, mash until you get the desired consistency.

Nutrition: Calories: 59 Fat: 0.2 g Carbohydrates 15.5 g Sugar 11.7 g Protein: 0.3 g Cholesterol 0 mg

CPSIA information can be obtained
at www.ICGtesting.com
Printed in the USA
BVHW050332080521
606757BV00010B/1339

9 781911 688266